Port Care

Roland Hennes · Gisela Müller
Editors

Port Care

Hygiene, Dressing Change, Monitoring, Complication Management

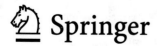 Springer

Editors
Roland Hennes
Clinic for General-, Visceral- and
Transplantation Surgery
Heidelberg University Hospital
Heidelberg, Germany

Gisela Müller
Surgical Clinic and Anaesthesiolgy Clinic
Heidelberg University Hospital
Heidelberg, Germany

ISBN 978-3-662-64493-5   ISBN 978-3-662-64494-2   (eBook)
https://doi.org/10.1007/978-3-662-64494-2

Preface

Port catheter systems have assumed a key role in the treatment of those patients in oncology and nutritional medicine. Effective cytotoxic combination therapies in oncological patients and sophisticated parenteral nutrition concepts have undergone a significant change. Safe implementation of these mostly intermittent therapies over long periods of time, avoidance or rather control of their complications require safe routes of administration. Port catheter systems are characterized by longevity, functional reliability, and low complication rates. They can remain in the body for years and demonstrate considerable advantages over temporary venous catheters such as PICC line or other central venous catheters. The easy handling of the port catheter systems by nurses and physicians indicates their application in the inpatient hospital sector, the outpatient clinic sector all the way to the home sector. The quality of life of patients increases due to a port catheter system, as freedom of movement and sporting activities such as swimming, hiking, walking, and many more are possible without restriction. Lower infection rates and fewer catheter problems compared to other central venous catheters enhance patient safety. Patients show a high acceptance regarding comfort and improved quality of life.

The proper installation of a port catheter system, correct use, and hygienic implementation in accordance with guidelines are fundamentally important processes in the handling of port catheter systems. In order to ensure this, expert knowledge and clear standards are required for the entire treatment process in compliance with hygiene guidelines, as well as responsible action by all those involved. The collegial and cooperative, interprofessional collaboration and communication of all participants, in all areas, is an essential aspect to ensure a long, complication-free course of treatment with a port catheter system. This textbook on port care is intended to be of support.

Mrs. Gisela Müller has been Head of Nursing Service in the Surgical Clinic at Heidelberg University Hospital since 2007. Together with her staff, she has made a significant contribution to realizing the goal of collegial cooperation and establishing a professional team of experts.

Based on her expertise as an oncology nurse, Barbara Fantl developed port training courses for all clinics at Heidelberg University and, together with Dr. Hennes, leads a team of port experts in order to responsibly implement competent care for port patients and to keep the development for improving care up to date.

This team of port experts also developed a nursing guideline for port patients, which became mandatory for all clinics of Heidelberg University Hospital.

Dr. Roland Hennes founded the world's first university center for port surgery in 2011, where more than 30,000 patients with port catheter systems have been advised and treated with port catheter systems since then. Several studies have been published on the topic of standardizing the treatment of patients with port catheter systems.

The textbook *"Ports"* was developed on the basis of more than 12,000 port implantations and extensive experience gained at the Heidelberg Port Center through close cooperation between nurses and physicians. Building on those results, this textbook is intended to comprehensively illustrate the evidence based, current state of port treatment and care and, at the same time, to be a practical book that provides the responsible nurses and physicians with the necessary knowledge to act quickly and unerringly incompetently treating their patients as well as advise and support them accordingly.

We would like to thank the team at Springer-Verlag, especially Ms. Sarah Busch and Ms. Ulrike Niesel, for their tireless support and expert supervision in making this textbook a reality.

The original version of the book has been revised. An erratum is available at https://doi.org/10.1007/978-3-662-60483-0_14

For reasons of better readability, we predominantly use the generic masculine in this book. This always implies both forms, thus including the female form.

Heidelberg, Germany   Gisela Müller
01.05.2020   Roland Hennes

Contents

1   Interdisciplinary Cooperation in Port Care   1
    Roland Hennes and Gisela Müller

2   Indications for a Port Catheter System, Basics of Port Surgery
    and Dealing with Complications from a Nursing Perspective   5
    Roland Hennes

3   Hygiene in Port Care   13
    Vanessa Eichel and Uwe Frank

4   Legal Aspects of Performing Port Puncture by Nurses: Delegation
    of Medical Activities   25
    Katja Maier

5   Expert Standard Port Care   31
    Barbara Fantl

6   Wound Care and Dressing Changes   45
    Barbara Fantl

7   Intraoperative and Postoperative Care of Port Patients   53
    Birgit Appelhoff and Lisa Moser

8   Special Features of Port Care for Oncological Patients   59
    Susann Eismann

9   Port Supply in Outpatient Care   65
    Halka Nehring and Anna Mindrup

10 Care of Special Patient Groups   79
    Julia Winkler, Debora Stern, Bianka Walter, and Damaris Weeber

11 Port Care for Children   87
    Heiko Riemke

12 **Documentation, Patient Counseling and Information** 95
    Margit Benz

13 **Evidence of Port Care** 103
    Reinhart T. Grundmann

Index 115

Roland Hennes and Gisela Müller

Summary In the implementation of necessary and appropriate treatment measures, port catheter systems have taken on a central role in modern oncology and nutritional medicine. The responsible and successful treatment of patients with a port catheter system poses particular requirements on nursing staff. First of all, we will explain what makes an implanted port catheter system so special and how this defines the demands for all professional groups and participants.

1.1   The Salient Feature of a Port Catheter System

A port catheter system consisting of a port chamber, a connecting mechanism and a port catheter is an access that remains in the body as an implant. This makes it accessible to anyone who punctures the port chamber with a suitable needle, establishing direct contact from the outside into the port chamber and thus into the bloodstream. In contrast, other implants, e.g., orthopaedic implants such as prostheses, only come into contact with the surgeon in terms of surgical implantation or explantation.

Puncture can in principle also lead to infection, which is why compliance with hygiene measures for sterile port catheter care is indispensable.

R. Hennes (✉)
Clinic for General-, Visceral- and Transplantation Surgery, Heidelberg University Hospital, Heidelberg, Germany
e-mail: roland.hennes@med.uni-heidelberg.de

G. Müller
Surgical Clinic and Anaesthesiolgy Clinic, Heidelberg University Hospital, Heidelberg, Germany
e-mail: gisela.mueller@med.uni-heidelberg.de

© Springer-Verlag GmbH Germany, part of Springer Nature 2022
R. Hennes, G. Müller (eds.), *Port Care*,
https://doi.org/10.1007/978-3-662-64494-2_1

1.2   Use and Evaluation of Port Catheter Systems

A port catheter system, nowadays ideally implanted as a high-pressure port system with a flow rate of 5 ml/s, can be used for many indications such as chemotherapy, nutritional therapy and pain therapy. In addition, the high-pressure port catheter systems offer the possibility of ensuring CT and MRI staging examinations through the administration of a contrast agent.

For the patient, a functioning port catheter system forms the basis for carrying out his necessary therapies and can be significant for his survival if vital medication and nutritional solutions have to be given. This also saves the patient the inconvenience and anxiety of constant frustrating punctures, e.g., on the forearms. Oncological patients in particular often no longer offer sufficient vein conditions on the forearm for a simple puncture. In addition, some chemotherapeutic agents may no longer be injected via peripheral veins, but only via a central venous catheter system.

Since port catheter systems are used in all oncological as well as nutritional medical facilities and also increasingly in radiological diagnostics, a large number of persons and professional groups are confronted with the handling of port catheter systems, which imposes a unique responsibility on them. It is essential that both medical and nursing staff who puncture a port catheter system receive standardized training and are thoroughly informed and instructed in the various systems (high-pressure port systems, double-chamber ports, ports for use in apheresis) as well as, for example, in the specificity of a port needle with a safety precaution. The editors overlook over 30,000 port patients treated at Heidelberg University Hospital over the last 15 years from 2005 to 2020.

Compliance with the legal aspects of port maintenance is equally important, as outlined in Chap. 5.

The initial puncture is the responsibility of the implanting physician, but this is usually done intraoperatively during the implantation of a port catheter system to check its functionality. In this respect, the initial puncture is basically already fulfilled by the surgical intervention. In the postoperative or outpatient sector, the puncture of a port catheter system is carried out on the instructions of a responsible physician.

The competent performance of puncturing a port catheter system requires consistently trained and educated personnel, including all physicians and nurses who perform this task. The expertise, which includes knowledge of materials such as port safety needles, skin disinfectant, composition of a port catheter system, length of time a port needle is in place, and many other important specific details, is essential for all who care for a port patient with his or her port catheter system. These specific points are covered in depth in the remaining chapters. The extraordinary importance of this expertise across all professions is reflected in the main problem of port catheter systems: namely, the risk of port infection with severe complications and costs.

1.3 Interdisciplinary Responsible Cooperation and Holistic Approach for the Port Patient

From all the experiences with thousands of patients, it is abundantly obvious that the appreciation and professional treatment of port patients should not only be improved, but transformed. Transformation in this context should mean that a real change in the treatment of port patients must take place. Practice and experience to this day show that only a few clinics or outpatient departments have standardized their procedures to the current level of knowledge (Fig. 1.1).

► Only a holistic approach—with the cooperation of all persons involved— guarantees successful treatment for the patient in the long run.

This means that in addition to the standardized training and information of physicians and nursing staff in the outpatient as well as in the clinical sector, the relatives and patients must also be well informed about the port catheter system. In particular, questions about the daily handling of the port catheter system (e.g. sports activities, personal hygiene, flushing, blocking the port catheter system) are very important for patients and relatives.

Within the topics of port care and the function of the port chamber, there is often the discrepancy that the responsible physicians are authorized to give instructions and are in charge of the treatment of the patient, but have far less practice and specific expertise than is already present and exercised by trained nurses. It is important to address this deficiency in the standardization of port care because it is here that pronounced discrepancies arise that can ultimately develop to the detriment of the port patient.

Fig. 1.1 Interdisciplinary cooperation. (From Heidelberg University Hospital, Port brochure "Interesting facts about your port" 2014)

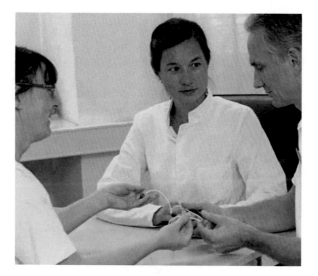

1.4   Conclusion

In summary, the following requirements must be met for competent and responsible treatment of port patients:

1. The standardized regular training of all professional groups involved—physicians as well as nursing staff—in the handling and performance of port puncture and care of the port catheter systems. This includes in particular the fulfilment of legal and hygienic requirements.
2. A holistic approach for the port patient with the selection and use of the right materials as well as sustainability in the quality of care through competent contact persons in the outpatient as well as in the clinical sector, where responsible nursing staff and physicians stand for competent treatment and patient satisfaction.

Indications for a Port Catheter System, Basics of Port Surgery and Dealing with Complications from a Nursing Perspective

2

Roland Hennes

Summary Patients who require a port catheter system for their treatment often come from the oncological and nutritional medicine sector. Here, the indications for the administration of chemotherapeutic agents, antibodies as well as nutritional solutions and other additive infusions and preparations are in the foreground. This chapter explains the indications for the insertion of a port catheter system, the possible locations as well as complications that can occur during implantation.

2.1 Indications

Patients who require a port catheter system for their treatment often come from the oncological and nutritional medicine sector. Here, the indications for the administration of chemotherapeutic agents, antibodies as well as nutritional solutions and other additive infusions and preparations are in the foreground. However, it should not be forgotten that the long-term administration of pain therapeutics can also be carried out via port catheter systems ("Ports", Hennes and Hofmann Springer 2016).

The structure of a port catheter system is shown in Fig. 2.1.

The development of the high-pressure ports, which are suitable for ensuring a flow rate of 5 ml/s via a pump, has given the port catheter system an additional function by allowing a contrast medium to be administered via the port for a CT or MRI examination. This saves patients with very poor peripheral vein conditions in particular the frustrating puncture of the forearms in order to administer the contrast medium.

The patient must show the radiologist his or her port passport showing that it is a high-pressure port catheter system so that the radiologist has the legal certainty that he or she can administer the contrast medium via the port.

R. Hennes (✉)
Clinic for General-, Visceral- and Transplantation Surgery, Heidelberg University Hospital, Heidelberg, Germany
e-mail: roland.hennes@med.uni-heidelberg.de

© Springer-Verlag GmbH Germany, part of Springer Nature 2022
R. Hennes, G. Müller (eds.), *Port Care*,
https://doi.org/10.1007/978-3-662-64494-2_2

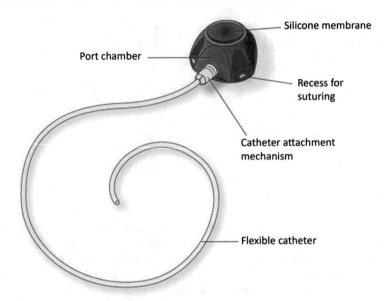

Fig. 2.1 Structure of a port catheter system (From Heidelberg University Hospital, Port brochure "Interesting facts about your port")

Port catheter systems that do not present the specification as a high-pressure port must not be used for contrast medium administration. The use of high-pressure port catheter systems is indispensable for modern oncological as well as nutritional medical treatment, since CT and MRI diagnostics with contrast medium administration are used for most patients.

Indications for a Port Catheter System
- Chemotherapy
- Nutritional solution
- Antibody administration
- Contrast agent administration for MRI/CT examination°
- Apharesis
- Dialysis pain therapy

2.2   Basics of the Port Operation

A nurse's or doctor's basic knowledge of how to approach a port patient includes being familiar with the principles of port surgery. This includes being aware of the possible locations of port catheter systems. The standard approach is to place port catheter systems thoracically, between the shoulder and chest muscles adjacent to

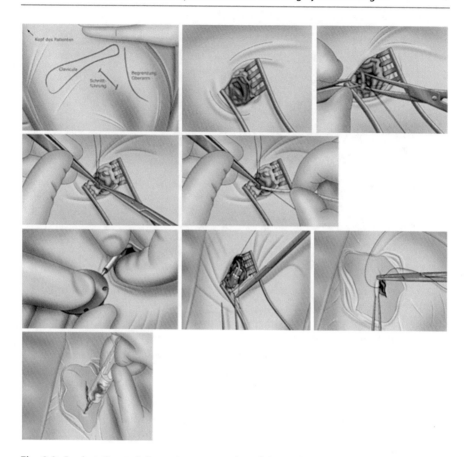

Fig. 2.2 Implantation technique via venae section of the cephalic vein in the Mohrenheim pit (Source: "Xope" Deutscher Ärzteverlag)

Mohrenheim's pit (see Fig. 2.2). This technique has proven to be a standardized access at the Universitätsklinik in Heidelberg (University Hospital in Heidelberg) and has also been positively assessed in several studies (Hennes and Hofmann "Ports" Springer 2016). A port catheter system is placed subcutaneously and ideally in such a way that it can be palpated as close as possible to the skin surface even in obese patients and can then also be punctured. In addition, it should be fixed, both the catheter in the soft tissue more precisely at the cephalic vein and the port chamber should be fixed with at least two fixation sutures on the pectoralis fascia. Otherwise, the port chamber may rotate and tilt, especially if the patient is very physically active immediately after port surgery (see Fig. 2.3). This is evident in situations where the silicone membrane of the port chamber is not accessible for puncture and one punctures, ohne onto the port body or the bottom of the port chamber, thus making port chamber puncture impossible. Such a port patient should be presented to the

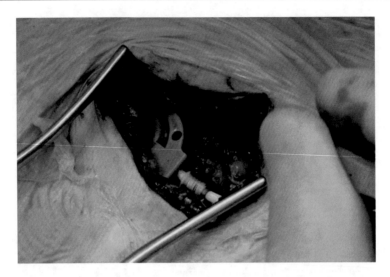

Fig. 2.3 Tilted port chamber in the absence of fixation (From Hennes and Hofmann 2016)

surgeon or a competent clinic, as there is an urgent indication for explantation or replacement of the port catheter system (Fischer et al. 2008).

Other locations for port catheter systems may be in the antecubital fossa or distal upper arm, with arm ports significantly limiting the patient's quality of life and freedom of movement. Here, nerve irritation, pressure discomfort and other port problems can occur, which can be associated with an increased risk of infection. In the case of prolonged thromboses and the impossibility of placing a port catheter system thoracically, the groin region offers another option (Hennes and Hofmann "Ports" Springer 2016).

A surgical procedure developed at Universitätsklinik Heidelberg (Heidelberg University Hospital) implements this by using a cross vein via an inguinal incision to place the port catheter. The catheter is then further tunneled and the port chamber is fixed externally to the tensor fascia lata in the proximal thigh area. Here, the port chamber for puncture is then located outside the groin region, which often has an increased density of germs, and the port chamber is located away from this on the thigh, where it can be very easily palpated and punctured.

▶ It is important to position the patient safely and correctly for all punctures of a port catheter system so that the port puncture can be performed safely. Here again, the hygiene guidelines for the performance must be absolutely adhered to (Chap. 3).

2.3 Dealing with Complications from the Nursing Perspective

Port chamber size can be quite challenging for the puncturing nurse or physician, as there is a great deal of variation in size from the smallest pediatric/baby ports to large lumen adult ports, which have an associated variation in puncture area (see Fig. 2.4).

▶ **Practical tip** If the port chamber can hardly or rather uncertainly be palpated in very obese patients, the port can be detected in the clinical setting with the aid of an ultrasound device and the safe puncture of the port chamber can be supported.

▶ It is always indispensable, as described in the following chapters, to key the port chamber safely and to select the correct port needle length.

In addition to inadequate fixation and tilting of the port chamber, kinking of the port catheter system is also one of the complications that can arise during port surgery (see Fig. 2.5).

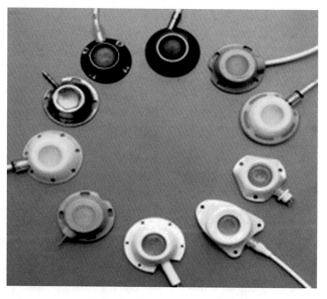

Fig. 2.4 Port chambers from different manufacturers with different puncture surfaces (From Heidelberg University Hospital, brochure "Interesting facts about your port" 2018)

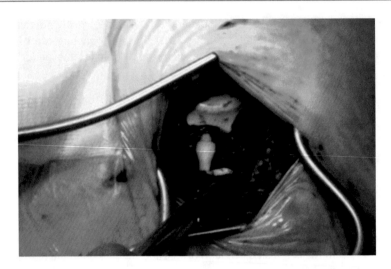

Fig. 2.5 Kinking of the port catheter (From Ports, Springer Hennes and Hofmann 2016)

These sometimes occur only after implantation, the functional test intraoperatively then shows that the port catheter system is operating properly, but during the first punctures the impracticability of the injection of fluid is discovered. This is rare, but can be observed again and again. Especially with silicone catheters, kinking can occur, which leads to complete occlusion of the port catheter and makes it impossible to be used.

▶   **Practical tip** This is important to know so that massive, unauthorised pressures via the injection syringes are not used here in an attempt to "force" the port catheter system into functioning (see Fig. 2.6). In such a case, the patient must be presented immediately to the operating surgeon or a competent expert, if possible.

To clarify such findings, fluoroscopy of the port catheter system with the administration of contrast medium is useful, in particular to rule out or detect leaks and extravasations (see Fig. 2.7).

As mentioned in the overview of indications in Sect. 2.1, port catheter systems are nowadays also used for apharesis. In this case, blood exchange takes place via large-lumen port catheters or so-called "apharesis ports". These show a normal port configuration and are accessed by a vertical puncture through the skin into the port chamber. An exception is a system on the market that can also be used for dialysis. This port catheter system requires an angular injection technique through the skin; the port needle must be passed at an angle of approximately 30–40°, depending on the constitution and configuration of this chamber. For this purpose, the manufacturer's instructions should be studied carefully before puncturing such an apharesis or dialysis port.

Fig. 2.6 Bulging of the silicone membrane from the port chamber due to the use of a 2 ml syringe with unauthorized pressure (From Ports, Springer Hennes and Hofmann 2016)

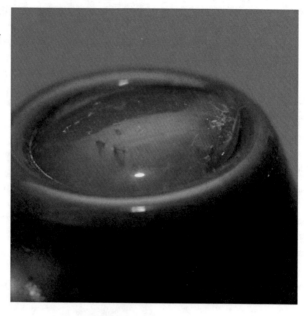

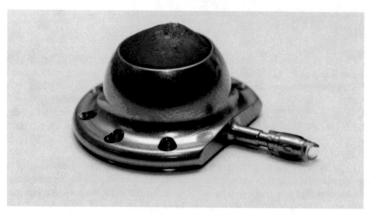

Fig. 2.7 Destroyed silicone membrane with observed extravasation of a 15-year-old port. (From Ports, Springer Hennes and Hofmann 2016)

Another special feature is the double chamber port. Here, two-port chambers can be palpated directly next to each other. This port is used for special indications and has a special design that prevents two infusions that have to be given at the same time from mixing. For this purpose, the catheter of the double chamber port has different outlets so that mixing of the substances cannot occur and, for example, precipitation of the infusion solutions is avoided. With a double chamber port, both chambers must be flushed and blocked.

▶ Port catheter systems can remain in the body for years and, with skilled and trained care, show the lowest complication rate for infection compared to other catheter systems, such as central venous or small catheters (Maki et al. 2006).

2.4 Conclusion

According to hygienic, legal and medically competent aspects, the nursing treatment of a port patient is a demanding activity that should only be carried out by trained personnel; this is also underlined by the guidelines of the Robert Koch Institute (RKI 2017). If problems occur during puncture of the port chamber, such as extravasation or impracticability in the case of occlusion, the patient should always be presented to a port expert (Fischer et al. 2008). The functionality of the port catheter system can be checked by fluoroscopy of the port catheter with a contrast medium. This provides information on the extent to which the catheter is passable, whether extravasations/leakages exist, and whether incorrect positions or kinks have occurred. Observation of the pathway, careful documentation and excellent and responsible care are the basis for complication-free and competent treatment of the port patient.

References

Fischer L, Knebel P, Schroder S, Bruckner T, Diener MK, Hennes R, Buhl K, Schmied B, Seiler CM (2008) Reasons for explantation of totally implantable access ports: a multivariate analysis of 385 consecutive patients. Ann Surg Oncol 15(4):1124–1129. https://doi.org/10.1245/s10434-007-9783-z

Hennes R, Hofmann HAF (2016) Ports, ISBN 978–3–662-436440-0. Springer, Heidelberg

Maki DG, Kluger DM, Crnich CJ (2006) The risk of bloodstream infection in adults with different intravascular devices: a systematic review of 200 published prospective studies. Mayo Clin Proc 81(9):1159–1171. https://doi.org/10.4065/81.9.1159

RKI (2017) Prävention von Infektionen, die von Gefäßkathetern ausgehen : Teil 1—Nichtgetunnelte zentralvenöse Katheter. Empfehlung der Kommission für Krankenhaushygiene und Infektionsprävention (KRINKO) beim Robert Koch-Institut. Bundesgesundheitsbl 60(2):171–206. https://doi.org/10.1007/s00103-016-2487-4

Hygiene in Port Care

3

Vanessa Eichel and Uwe Frank

Summary Infection is the most frequent complication of a port system and, in addition to antibiotics and port explantation, can mean intensive care requirements and be life-threatening for the patient. This illustrates the high importance of hygiene in handling the port. Disinfection can only be successful in conjunction with all other appropriate hygiene measures. The basis for hygiene in handling ports is the so-called standard or basic hygiene. This includes hand hygiene, protective equipment, behavior when coughing, sneezing and blowing one's nose, cleaning/disinfection of the patient environment, correct preparation and safe injection technique.

3.1 Basic Principles of Hygiene

The basis for hygiene in handling ports is the so-called standard or basic hygiene. This includes hand hygiene, protective equipment, behavior when coughing, sneezing and blowing one's nose, cleaning/disinfection of the patient environment, correct preparation and safe injection technique.

3.1.1 Hand Disinfection

VAH-listed, alcohol-based **hand disinfectants** with refatting substances are used for hand disinfection (e.g. Sterillium® classic pure). In case of outbreaks caused by non-enveloped viruses, such as noro-, polio- and adenoviruses, compounds with enhanced virucidal activity and a corresponding spectrum of activity are recommended (e.g. desderman® pure, Sterillium® virugard, Softa-Man® acute). The exposure time depends on the preparation and the indication.

V. Eichel · U. Frank (✉)
Section for Hospital and Environmental Hygiene, Heidelberg University Hospital, Heidelberg, Germany
e-mail: vanessa.eichel@med.uni-heidelberg.de; uwe.frank@med.uni-heidelberg.de

© Springer-Verlag GmbH Germany, part of Springer Nature 2022
R. Hennes, G. Müller (eds.), *Port Care*,
https://doi.org/10.1007/978-3-662-64494-2_3

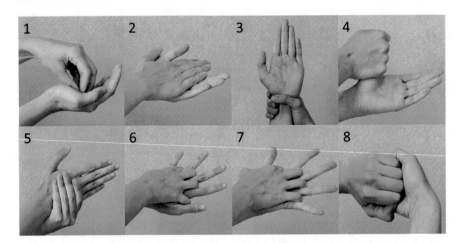

Fig. 3.1 Steps of hand disinfection. A liquid level of disinfectant is placed in each palm and the fingertips are dipped into it in a rotating motion (1). Then the disinfectant is spread on the hands up to at least the wrist (2, 3). In particular, the thumb (4), back of the hand and fingers (5), spaces between the fingers (6, 7) and nail folds (8) are rubbed in. (Source: Section for Hospital Hygiene of Heidelberg University Hospital)

A distinction is made between hygienic and surgical hand disinfection; the latter is not discussed here. Hygienic hand disinfection is performed for the five WHO indications (before and after patient contact, before aseptic activities, after contact with infectious material, after contact with the patient's immediate environment) as well as before and after the use of gloves and before entering a ward or department (Fig. 3.1) (RKI 2016).

▶ **Practical tip** The hands are completely wetted with 3–5 ml (at least 2 strokes) of disinfectant and rubbed until dry. Particular attention should be paid to fingertips and thumbs, as these areas are most frequently forgotten. The procedure according to standardized movement steps is not obligatory, but is suitable for learning the technique. The standard application time is usually 30 s.

3.1.2 Skin Disinfection

VAH-listed, alcohol-based **skin disinfectants** are used for skin disinfection. A distinction is made between skin disinfectants with and without an additional remanent (long-lasting) active ingredient. Skin disinfectants without remanence, such as Cutasept® and Softasept®, are indicated, for example, prior to punctures, blood sampling, injections and manipulation at connection sites. Substances with retentive additives, e.g., octenidine in Octeniderm®, chlorhexidine in Skinsept® and

PVP iodine in Braunoderm®, are always used if the skin barrier remains broken for a prolonged period of time. This is the case during the placement of vascular catheters and also during port puncture. The exposure time varies depending on the preparation, indication and sebaceous gland or fat content of the skin area (RKI 2017).

3.1.3   Surface Disinfection

Surface disinfection is carried out with a VAH-listed **surface disinfectant**. Disinfection of a surface or an object is indicated, for example, before and after use, especially before aseptic activities, after contamination, when changing patients and at regular intervals (RKI 2011) (Table 3.1).

Table 3.1 Overview of disinfectants commonly used in clinical facilities

Application	Indications	Products	How to use
Hygienic hand disinfection	Five WHO indications, before and after use of gloves, before entering a ward or department. Standard preparation	Sterillium® classic pure Skinman® clear	Wet hands completely with 3–5 ml (2 strokes) of disinfectant and rub until dry. Pay particular attention to fingertips and thumbs (EWZ 30 s).
	Five WHO indications, before and after use of gloves, before entering a ward or department. Unenveloped viruses e.g. noroviruses, adenoviruses, outbreaks	desderman® pure Sterillium® virugard Softa-Man® acute	Wet hands completely with 3–5 ml (2 strokes) of disinfectant and rub until dry. Pay particular attention to fingertips and thumbs (EWZ 30–60 s).
Skin disinfection	Before injections and punctures	Cutasept® Softasept® Kodan® Poly-Alcohol Skin®	Spray, wipe, spray (EWZ 30 s)
	Before invasive procedures with a particular risk of infection (e.g. before insertion of vascular catheters, port puncture, joint punctures)	Octeniderm® Skinsept® Braunoderm®	Spray 2 times and wipe sterile, spray again and allow to absorb (EWZ 2–10 min according to manufacturer's instructions)
Surface disinfection	Before and after use, in particular before aseptic activities, after contamination, when changing patients and at regular intervals	Incidin® Plus Bacillol® AF	Wipe disinfection with gloves for self-protection

EWZ Exposure time

3.2   Infection Routes of Port Catheters and the Importance of Hygiene

Infection is the most common complication of a port system and the most common reason for port explantation (Fischer et al. 2008; Narducci et al. 2011). The overall incidence of port infection diverges due to patient-specific factors and type of infusions, but hygiene measures can influence the infection rate. It has been reported to range from 0.8% to 10% (Lebeaux et al. 2014; Teichgraber et al. 2011). However, compared to other vascular catheter systems, the infection frequency of ports is considered to be lower, especially with long-term use (Maki et al. 2006).

When foreign material, such as a catheter, is inserted into the vascular system, it is covered with a fibrin layer within seconds. After microbial contamination, biofilms can form on the catheter wall, which severely impair the effect of antibiotics used. Almost all pathogens relevant to vascular catheters are capable of forming a biofilm (Donlan 2001). It is therefore essential to minimize contamination of the port by appropriate hygiene measures.

Possible routes of infection from ports are:

- the implantation
- the bloodstream hematogenous
- the handling of the port (skin flora)

3.2.1   Implantation

If the port is implanted by an experienced implanter in compliance with standard hygiene in the operating room, the infection rate is low. In a study of over 2270 port patients, infections occurred as an early complication in approximately 1.5% of ports within $\leq$30 days of implantation compared to approximately 3% after >30 days (Busch et al. 2017).

3.2.2   Bloodstream Hematogenous

Pathogens that circulate transitorily in the vascular system can adhere to the port and lead to a hematogenous port infection (Lebeaux et al. 2014). This proportion is low and can hardly be influenced by hygiene measures (Anaissie et al. 1995).

3.2.3   Handling the Port (Skin Flora)

In vascular catheter infections, pathogens most frequently enter from the outside along extra- and intraluminal routes. The skin flora of the patient and staff can be introduced into the hub through the spread of germs, e.g., if hygiene rules are disregarded, and lead to intraportal or intraluminal colonisation. This can manifest clinically as intermittent bacteremia with elevated temperature after use of the port or as sepsis. However, skin germs can also be transported through the perforation site of the skin, e.g., by capillary action, electrostatic forces, diffusion or when the port is pierced after inadequate skin disinfection, and colonise the outside of the port, which, depending on the depth, leads to a "pocket infection" or "exit site infection", which always requires port explantation (Eggimann and Pittet 2002; Mermel 2011).

Pathogen

The most common pathogens of port infections are *Staphylococcus epidermidis, Staphylococcus aureus, Candidae spp.* and, increasingly, gram-negative bacteria (Table 3.2) (Lebeaux et al., 2014).

Skin Disinfection

The use of an alcohol-based skin disinfectant with octenidine or chlorhexidine additive is recommended by the RKI (category IB, II). The insertion of a port needle, like the insertion of a CVC, can lead to a long-lasting disruption of the skin barrier by a catheter system. Therefore, a remanent skin disinfectant should be used here as well. In a study, a chlorhexidine additive is superior to a PVP-iodine additive for gram-positive pathogens, but the total number of port-associated infections could not be significantly reduced (Kao et al. 2014).

The RKI does not state whether spraying alone and waiting for the exposure time is sufficient or whether dirt, sweat and skin grease should be removed initially by spraying and wiping with a sterile swab (RKI 2011). At the Port Centre of Heidelberg University Hospital, the decision was made in favour of the latter procedure, as it only involves an additional effort of a few seconds.

Table 3.2 Microorganisms ($n = 103$) isolated from 97 port-related infections (Mod. according to (Lebeaux et al. 2014)

Pathogen	n (%)
Gram positive bacteria	59 (57)
Coagulase-negative staphylococci	30 (29)
Staphylococcus aureus	26 (25)
Enterococcus faecalis	1 (1)
Streptococcus pneumoniae	2 (2)
Gram-negative bacteria	42 (41)
Pseudomonas aeruginosa	9 (9)
Escherichia coli	9 (9)
Klebsiella spp.	7 (7)
Enterobacter cloacae	8 (8)
Acinetobacter baumannii	3 (3)
Serratia marcescens	3 (3)
Pantoea spp.	1 (1)
Aeromonas spp.	1 (1)
Proteus mirabilis	1 (1)
Yeast-like fungi	2 (2)

Blocking the Port

If the port system is filled with a substance that is to remain in the port catheter until the next application, this is called a block. Blocking is used for infection and thrombosis prevention and as a therapeutic option. A comprehensive meta-analysis by Goossens compared the preventive agents used to block vascular catheters with NaCl 0.9%. Saline blocking was found to be non-inferior to heparin blocking. Ethanol and antibiotic solutions should only be used after consideration and taking into account the respective side effects (Goossens 2015). Taurolidine block was able to reduce the catheter-related infection rate in a meta-analysis with small numbers of cases, while the thrombosis rate was not influenced (Liu et al. 2013).

Needle Change

There is no sufficient evidence on the frequency of needle changes (category III) (RKI 2017). At the Port Center of Heidelberg University Hospital, it has proven effective to schedule needle changes every 5 days, as this ensures that a lying time of 7 days is not exceeded under any circumstances, even in the event of delays.

Personnel Conditions

Several studies have demonstrated that personnel resources and qualifications of the staff performing the procedure have a significant impact on vascular catheter infection rates (Needleman et al. 2002; Safdar et al. 2002). The frequency of port operation correlates with the likelihood of infection (Lebeaux et al. 2014). Therefore, incorrect attempts to pierce the port should be reduced, for example, by training with model-based exercises on the model. In rare cases, a non-sterile infusion solution can also lead to an infection of the port system.

▶   **Practical tip** The establishment of a binding standard for the handling of
    port systems as well as training and education for all executing
    employees have proven themselves in practice and are absolutely
    recommended.

3.3   Recommendations of the RKI

The following recommendations of the Commission for Hospital Hygiene and Infection Prevention of the Robert Koch Institute were summarised by the German Society for Haematology and Medical Oncology (Uhrig 2015). The recommendation grades of the Robert Koch Institute are explained in Table 3.3.

- Training programme for nurses and doctors based on written nursing instructions (IB)
- Implantation of port systems under aseptic conditions in the operating or procedure room (IB)
- Hygienic hand disinfection before or after bandage replacement (IB)

Table 3.3 Levels of recommendation of the Commission for Hospital Hygiene and Infection Prevention of the Robert Koch Institute (RKI 2017)

Category	Definition
IA	This recommendation is based on well-designed systematic reviews or single high-quality randomized controlled trials
IB	This recommendation is based on clinical or high-quality epidemiological studies and rigorous, plausible and comprehensible theoretical derivations
II	This recommendation is based on indicative studies/investigations and rigorous, plausible and comprehensible theoretical derivations
III	Measures on whose effectiveness there is insufficient or contradictory evidence, therefore a recommendation is not possible
IV	Requirements, measures and procedures to be observed by generally applicable legislation

- Disinfection of the puncture site with skin disinfectant, taking into account the exposure time (IB)
- Bandage replacement using a non-touch technique or sterile gloves (IB)
- If necessary, clean the insertion site with sterile NaCl solution 0.9% and sterile swab (IB)
- Application of antiseptics—preferably alcohol-based skin disinfectants—to the insertion site during bandage replacement (II)
- No use of ointments or gels for transparent dressings (IB)
- Non-pierced port catheters do not need a dressing (IB)
- The puncture site is to be disinfected over a large area, observing the prescribed exposure time of the disinfectant (IB)
- Sterile gloves must be worn for the puncture, which involves palpation and fixation of the port chamber between the palpating fingers (IB)
- Only suitable special cannulas may be used (IB)
- Aseptic connection of the infusion system (IB)
- No recommendation on the maximum duration of use of port needles (III)
- Unmanageable complications require removal of the port system. Immediate removal of the port system in case of damage or dislocation (IB)

3.4 Handling the Port System

The procedure for handling the port system described in this chapter was developed at the Portzentrum des Universitätsklinikum Heidelberg (Port Center of Heidelberg University Hospital) in cooperation with the Section for Hospital and Environmental Hygiene and has proven to be a binding standard in practice. The hygienic handling of the port system was implemented by the authors using video technology (http://blue-wing-pictures.com/hygiene-tutorial/).

3.4.1   Monitoring of the Port Catheter

- Documentation of the implantation site
- Secure fixation of the port needle
- Daily inspection of the position of the port needle, the port environment and the dressing. Palpation is not necessary with transparent dressings and should be avoided
- If not used, flush the port every 3 months exclusively with at least 10 ml NaCl 0.9% using the push-and-go technique

3.4.2   Change of Dressing of the Port Catheter

- Transparent film dressings can be left in place until the needle is changed (maximum 7 days), provided there are no signs of infection. Change the dressing if it becomes soaked, soiled or loose
- Dressing changes should be performed using a non-touch technique or sterile gloves
- Avoid unnecessary palpations/manipulations
- Ensure safe post-fixation of the infusion system

3.4.3   Puncture of the Port Catheter

3.4.4   Material

- Hand disinfectant
- Skin disinfectant (with added octenidine or chlorhexidine)
- Surface disinfectant
- Sterile cloth
- Mouthguard
- Non-sterile gloves
- Sterile gloves
- 4 packs of sterile compresses
- 2 syringes à 10 ml NaCl 0.9%, sterile packaging
- Port needle (patient-specific, recommendation see port ID card or last patient documentation)
- Sterile cap
- Drop box
- Transparent foil bandage and plaster for fixation
- Deposit

▶   **Practical tip** It is essential to use an alcohol-based skin disinfectant with
     a remanent additive for skin disinfection during port puncture.
- Hygienic hand disinfection
- Greeting and questioning of the patient. Positioning and undressing the patient in preparation for the puncture
- Put on mouth guard and non-sterile gloves
- Palpation of the port chamber and assessment of the puncture site
- Wipe-disinfect the tray with a surface disinfectant
- Spread sterile drape on tray and drop sterile material onto drape. Provide disinfectant, sterile compresses and plasters next to it
- Disinfection of the puncture area with a skin disinfectant
- Disinfect the puncture area extensively and wipe it sterile 2 times each
- Disinfect the puncture area again and allow to absorb
- Remove non-sterile gloves during the exposure time, perform hygienic hand disinfection and put on sterile gloves
- Venting the 3-way stopcock with NaCl 0.9%
- Connection of the 3-way stopcock with the port needle and venting of the entire tubing system with NaCl 0.9%
- Remove needle guard
- Palpation of the port chamber and fixation of the port with two fingers
- Have patient look in the opposite direction
- Hold the port needle securely and puncture perpendicular to the port membrane until the needle stops
- Open the clamp of the port needle
- Aspiration test, if not possible, only rinse carefully with 10 ml NaCl 0.9% without resistance
- Rinse carefully with at least 20 ml NaCl 0.9% using the push-and-go technique
- Turn over the 3-way stopcock, remove the syringe and put on the cap without touching the areas to be connected (non-touch technique)
- Sticking the port needle onto the skin (in case of adhesive port needles) and sealing with transparent foil
- To fix the extension of the 3-way stopcock or similar, plaster strips are applied at a sufficient distance from the puncture site

3.4.5 Administering Infusions

- Hygienic hand disinfection
- Put on non-sterile gloves
- Place sterile compress underneath to avoid contact of the connection site with the skin
- Disinfect the cap of the 3-way stopcock with a skin disinfectant
- Remove cap and spray into the cone
- Allow to act and shake out alcohol residues over the sterile compress

- Connection with the infusion system in non-touch technique and flipping of the 3-way stopcock

Disconnections are to be reduced to an absolute minimum. After each disconnection, a new sterile cap must be applied. If several therapeutic substances are administered, flush intermediately with 10 ml NaCl 0.9%. Always rinse with at least 20 ml NaCl 0.9% after the end of the infusion.

3.4.6   Blood Collection/Blood Transfusion (Only after Risk Assessment)

Blood sampling and transfusions from vascular catheters should be avoided. If, after weighing the risk, a blood sample or transfusion is nevertheless to be taken via the port, the following procedure is recommended:

- Using a 19 gauge port needle
- Hygienic hand disinfection
- Put on non-sterile gloves
- Place sterile compress underneath to avoid contact of the catheter stroke with the skin
- Disinfect the cap of the 3-way stopcock with a skin disinfectant and open it
- Aspirate and discard at least 10 ml of blood
- After blood collection or transfusion, rinse with at least 20 ml (50 ml is optimal) NaCl 0.9%

3.4.7   Removal of the Port Needle

- Hygienic hand disinfection
- Flush the port with 10 ml NaCl 0.9%
- Put on non-sterile gloves
- Fixation of the port with two fingers, grasping the port needle and pulling it
- Safely dispose of the port needle in the designated dropbox
- Skin disinfection
- During the exposure time, remove gloves and perform hygienic hand disinfection
- Care of the puncture site with sterile wound plaster

3.4.8   Documentation

The person performing the procedure documents in the patient file and port passport

- the position, size of the port needle and the date of insertion of the port needle
- the regression of the port

- the maintenance of the port
- the specifics and complications
- the removal of the port needle
- the flushing of the port when not in use

3.5 Evidence/Infection Management

For further evidence and infection management, see Chap. 13.

3.6 Conclusion

Infection is the most frequent complication of a port system and, in addition to antibiotics and port explantation, can mean intensive care requirements and be life-threatening for the patient. This illustrates the high importance of hygiene in handling the port. Disinfection can only be successful in conjunction with all other appropriate hygiene measures. Therefore, the establishment of a binding standard for the handling of port systems as well as training for all executing staff members is necessary in order to minimize the part of port infections that could be avoided by appropriate hygienic measures. This requires good cooperation between all professional groups involved as well as the inclusion of the patient and, if necessary, the relatives, so that everyone can contribute to infection prevention and assume responsibility.

References

Anaissie E, Samonis G, Kontoyiannis D, Costerton J, Sabharwal U, Bodey G, Raad I (1995) Role of catheter colonization and infrequent hematogenous seeding in catheter-related infections. Eur J Clin Microbiol Infect Dis 14(2):134–137. https://doi.org/10.1007/bf02111873

Busch JD, Vens M, Mahler C, Herrmann J, Adam G, Ittrich H (2017) Complication rates observed in silicone and polyurethane catheters of totally implanted central venous access devices implanted in the upper arm. J Vasc Interv Radiol 28(8):1177–1183. https://doi.org/10.1016/j.jvir.2017.04.024

Donlan RM (2001) Biofilms and device-associated infections. Emerg Infect Dis 7(2):277

Eggimann P, Pittet D (2002) Overview of catheter-related infections with special emphasis on prevention based on educational programs. Clin Microbiol Infect 8(5):295–309. https://doi.org/10.1046/j.1469-0691.2002.00467.x

Fischer L, Knebel P, Schroder S, Bruckner T, Diener MK, Hennes R, Seiler CM (2008) Reasons for explantation of totally implantable access ports: a multivariate analysis of 385 consecutive patients. Ann Surg Oncol 15(4):1124–1129. https://doi.org/10.1245/s10434-007-9783-z

Goossens GA (2015) Flushing and locking of venous catheters: available evidence and evidence deficit. Nurs Res Pract 2015:985686. https://doi.org/10.1155/2015/985686

Kao H-F, Chen I-C, Hsu C, Chang S-Y, Chien S-F, Chen Y-C, Yeh K-H (2014) Chlorhexidine for the prevention of bloodstream infection associated with totally implantable venous ports in patients with solid cancers. Support Care Cancer 22(5):1189–1197. https://doi.org/10.1007/s00520-013-2071-5

Lebeaux D, Fernandez-Hidalgo N, Chauhan A, Lee S, Ghigo JM, Almirante B, Beloin C (2014) Management of infections related to totally implantable venous-access ports: challenges and perspectives. Lancet Infect Dis 14(2):146–159. https://doi.org/10.1016/s1473-3099(13)70266-4

Liu Y, Zhang AQ, Cao L, Xia HT, Ma JJ (2013) Taurolidine lock solutions for the prevention of catheter-related bloodstream infections: a systematic review and meta-analysis of randomized controlled trials. PLoS One 8(11):e79417. https://doi.org/10.1371/journal.pone.0079417

Maki DG, Kluger DM, Crnich CJ (2006) The risk of bloodstream infection in adults with different intravascular devices: a systematic review of 200 published prospective studies. Mayo Clin Proc 81(9):1159–1171. https://doi.org/10.4065/81.9.1159

Mermel LA (2011) What is the predominant source of intravascular catheter infections? Clin Infect Dis 52(2):211–212. https://doi.org/10.1093/cid/ciq108

Narducci F, Jean-Laurent M, Boulanger L, El Bedoui S, Mallet Y, Houpeau JL, Fournier C (2011) Totally implantable venous access port systems and risk factors for complications: a one-year prospective study in a cancer Centre. Eur J Surg Oncol 37(10):913–918. https://doi.org/10.1016/j.ejso.2011.06.016

Needleman J, Buerhaus P, Mattke S, Stewart M, Zelevinsky K (2002) Nurse-staffing levels and the quality of care in hospitals. N Engl J Med 346(22):1715–1722. https://doi.org/10.1056/nejmsa012247

RKI (2011) Anforderungen an die Hygiene bei Punktionen und Injektionen. Bundesgesundheitsbl 54:1135–1144. https://doi.org/10.1007/s00103-011-1352-8

RKI (2016) Händehygiene in Einrichtungen des Gesundheitswesens. Bundesgesundheitsbl 59(9):1189–1220. https://doi.org/10.1007/s00103-016-2416-6

RKI (2017) Prävention von Infektionen, die von Gefäßkathetern ausgehen: Teil 1—Nichtgetunnelte zentralvenöse Katheter Empfehlung der Kommission für Krankenhaushygiene und Infektionsprävention (KRINKO) beim Robert Koch-Institut. Bundesgesundheitsbl 60(2):171–206. https://doi.org/10.1007/s00103-016-2487-4

Safdar N, Kluger DM, Maki DG (2002) A review of risk factors for catheter-related bloodstream infection caused by percutaneously inserted, noncuffed central venous catheters: implications for preventive strategies. Medicine (Baltimore) 81(6):466–479

Teichgraber UK, Pfitzmann R, Hofmann HA (2011) Central venous port systems as an integral part of chemotherapy. Dtsch Arztebl Int 108(9):147–153, quiz 154. https://doi.org/10.3238/arztebl.2011.0147

Uhrig M (2015) Portkatheter. Deutsche Gesellschaft für Hämatologie und Medizinische Onkologie e. V. https://www.onkopedia.com/de/onkopedia-p/guidelines/portkatheter/@@view/pdf/index.pdf

Legal Aspects of Performing Port Puncture by Nurses: Delegation of Medical Activities

Katja Maier

Summary There are no specific legal regulations on the performance of port punctures by nurses. The general legal situation regarding the delegation of medical activities to nursing staff is currently unclear and not conclusively regulated. A uniform implementation of the delegation of certain medical activities is currently to be tested by the Heilkunde Transfer Directive[1] (HÜR) within the framework of pilot projects.

4.1 Highly Personalized Service Provision and Delegation

The physician does not have to provide every service personally, as is stipulated by the principle of personal provision of services. Medical services can be transferred to non-medical staff, at least this is approved by the legislator. This also applies to the performance of port punctures by trained nursing staff. However, the preconditions for the delegation of medical services to nursing staff are decisively shaped by the old understanding of the personal provision of services by the physician. The responsibility of the physician for the performance of the medical service and the merely supportive assistance of the nursing staff represent the common relationship between the two professional groups.

There are numerous legal bases for the personal provision of medical services. They are found in the contract law on services (§ 613 of the German Civil Code-BGB), in the Code of Social Law V (§ 15 Para. 1 S. 1 SGB V), in the professional

---

[1] "Guideline on the determination of medical activities for transfer to professionals of geriatric and nursing care for the independent practice of medicine within the framework of model projects according to § 63 para. 3 c SGB".

K. Maier (✉)
Heidelberg University Hospital, Heidelberg, Germany
e-mail: Katja.Maier@med.uni-heidelberg.de

© Springer-Verlag GmbH Germany, part of Springer Nature 2022
R. Hennes, G. Müller (eds.), *Port Care*,
https://doi.org/10.1007/978-3-662-64494-2_4

law (§ 19 Para. 1 S. 1 Musterberufsordnung-Ä-MBO-Ä), the contract physician law (§ 32 Para. 1 S. 1 Zulassungsordnung für Vertragsärzte, § 15 Abs. 1 S. 1 Bundesmantelvertrag-Ärzte) as well as in billing and remuneration regulations of medical services (§ 4 Abs. 2 Gebührenordnung für Ärzte, § 17 Abs. 1 Krankenhausentgeltgesetz).

Shaped by this structure, the performance of medical tasks by qualified and, if necessary, additionally trained nursing staff is permissible according to developed case law. Provided that the physician has ordered the activity, spot-checked the quality of the performance and is within call range, so that monitoring remains possible.[2] Furthermore, the documentation of the order is required for evidence and control purposes (§ 10 MBO-Ä and § 630h para. 3 BGB). The assessment of whether the non-medical staff is sufficiently qualified (subjective requirement) is the responsibility of the physician. The actual know-how of the staff member is decisive here. For port puncture by nursing staff, according to the German Medical Association, the administration of medication or infusion via a port can be delegated, depending on the medication to be administered and the qualification of the nurse; the initial intravenous administration of a medication, on the other hand, cannot.[3]

Which activities can be delegated under these conditions is not clearly specified or defined by the legislator. There is only a core area of medical activities that cannot be delegated and is reserved for the physician alone. According to the German Medical Association, this includes "anamnesis, indication, examination of the patient including invasive and diagnostic services, making a diagnosis, informing and advising the patient, deciding on therapy and carrying out invasive therapies including the core services of surgical interventions".[4] Activities are also to be performed by the physician in a highly personal capacity if their "difficulty, danger or unpredictability"[5] requires the physician's expertise. The higher the physician therefore assesses the health risk for the patient (objective requirement), the more the activity lies within the physician's area of responsibility. The physician must therefore always make a case-by-case assessment.

As a legal consequence, the hospital, as the service provider, is held contractually liable under the treatment contract with the patient as the service provider (§§ 630a ff. BGB in conjunction with §§ 280 Para. 1, 278 BGB) and can internally take recourse against the doctor or nurse. Due to the employer's duty of care and an existing liability insurance of the facility, such action is usually not necessary. Tortious liability for damages and compensation for pain and suffering can also

---

[2] Guidelines of the German Medical Association on "Possibilities and Limits of Delegation of Medical Services" via www.bundesaerztekammer.de, as of 29.08.2008; Katzenmeier in: Laufs/ Katzenmeier/Lipp, Ärztetrecht, 7th edition, 2015, X. Arztfehler und Haftpflicht, marginal no. 57.

[3] Guidelines of the German Medical Association on "Possibilities and Limits of Delegation of Medical Services" via www.bundesaerztekammer.de, as of 29.08.2008.

[4] Guidelines of the German Medical Association on "Possibilities and Limits of Delegation of Medical Services" via www.bundesaerztekammer.de, as of 29.08.2008.

[5] OLG Dresden, judgement of 24.07.2008 – file number 4 U 1857/07, BeckRS 2008, 17814, beck-online.

affect the physician if the delegated activity was demonstrably performed incorrectly or a task was delegated that is subject to the physician's prerogative (§ 823 Para. 1 BGB in conjunction with § 831 BGB). Liability is excluded if the physician can prove that the nurse was carefully selected and supervised. Since the regulation affects the acting staff member personally, the nurse can be made responsible besides for own obligation injury (§ 823 exp. 1 BGB). If the physician is proven to have violated his duties in the delegation, criminal liability for bodily injury, homicide, failure to render assistance or billing fraud may be added.

4.2   Problematic Points of the Current Legal Situation

The limits of delegable activities are therefore difficult to define and regularly lead to case-by-case decisions by the courts. These cannot be transferred to every case and do not provide sufficient legal certainty. Rather, the current legal situation gives rise to difficult questions of demarcation between the nursing and medical professions. In the absence of legislative guidelines, there is also uncertainty about the question of which medication can be delegated to qualified nursing staff for port puncture. The following further problem areas exist with regard to delegation to non-medical staff:

4.2.1   Patient's Consent

The scope of consent is found in the completed treatment contract. As a rule, it extends to treatment by qualified staff only. If the doctor delegates the activity to non-qualified nursing staff or assigns a task that cannot be delegated, the patient's consent to the treatment is lacking. In the absence of justifiable consent by the patient, this can lead to criminal liability of the doctor or nurse for bodily harm.

4.2.2   Billability of the Service

If the physician does not personally provide a medical service within the framework of elective physician agreements, this can lead to billing problems (§ 4 Para. 2 GoÄ and § 17 Para. 1 KHEntG) as well as to criminal proceedings for billing fraud (§ 263 StGB). The physician may delegate a service to non-medical personnel if the activity is performed under his supervision according to professional instructions (§ 4 Para. 2 GoÄ); however, more than a careful selection and supervision by the elective physician must take place.[6] According to case law, a so-called "personal imprint" is required.[7] Accordingly, the control of the treatment must be incumbent

---

[6]Spickhoff, Seibl: Die Erstattung ärztlicher Leistung bei Delegation an nichtärztliches Personal, NZS (2008, p. 59).

[7]OLG Celle, judgment of 15.06.2015 – file number 1 U 98/14, BeckRS 2015, 12522, beck-online.

on the physician. On the other hand, it is owed to the patient's will and the patient's safety that services of a non-medical employee are partly regarded as non-billable elective physician services.[8]

4.2.3 Efficiency

The parallel responsibility of physicians and nursing staff due to inadequately delimited areas of responsibility promotes inefficient work structures and unnecessarily consumed resources. The workload of physicians cannot be reduced in this way by the continuous monitoring duties.

4.3 Specialization of Care

In order to solve the difficulties of demarcation and to do justice to modern structures, the construct of personal service provision by the physician must be further developed. There is a need for autonomous areas of responsibility for non-physician staff that lead to a clear demarcation of responsibilities and facilitate cooperation. The specialization of nursing staff through additional qualifications can enable a clear distribution and resolve uncertainties.

It is not only the increasing complexity of medical treatments that calls for the specialization and further training of nursing staff; the so-called "nursing shortage" could also be counteracted by additional qualifications for nursing staff. Relief for doctors is only a positive effect if qualified non-medical staff carry out tasks assigned to them independently and on their own responsibility. Specific further training of nursing staff and the emergence of new occupational fields can create incentives to take up the nursing profession. A useful division of labour and simplified procedures can lead to greater job satisfaction and optimization of work processes. Furthermore, increasing specialization leads to greater job security in the nursing sector.[9]

4.4 Approach to Structuring—The Health Care Transfer Directive

The HÜR is an attempt to redistribute traditional roles among other modern approaches (case management) and to create legal clarity. It specifies which medical activities can be transferred to nurses and geriatric nurses and which supplementary qualifications a nurse must have in order to be allowed to transfer a medical activity

---

[8] At least according to Spickhoff, Seibl: Die Erstattung ärztlicher Leistung bei Delegation an nichtärztliches Personal, NZS (2008, p. 60).

[9] Spickhoff, Seibl: Die Erstattung ärztlicher Leistung bei Delegation an nichtärztliches Personal, NZS (2008, p. 57).

for independent practice. As early as 2008, the Federal Joint Committee (G-BA) was commissioned by the legislature to adopt a guideline on the transfer of medical activities to nurses for the elderly and the sick within the framework of the Nursing Care Further Development Act. The HÜR was then adopted by the G-BA on 20.10.2011 and came into force on March 22, 2012. With this, the G-BA created the basis for testing the transfer of medical activities within so-called model projects. The aim of the guideline is the independent and autonomous exercise of curative activities by nurses without medical supervision (Section 2 (2) HÜR).

In order to be transferred to a nurse, the latter must be certified (§§ 1, 2 KrPflG). In addition to the original learning content, extended competences for the practice of medicine must be taught (§ 4 Para. 7 KrPflG). The extended training content is to be defined by the training schools in such a way that the medical practice can ultimately be exercised.

By transferring the activity to the nurse, the latter is not only responsible for the performance in professional, economic and legal terms, but also has the authority to decide whether and to what extent the practice of medicine is medically indicated (§ 2 Para. 2 HÜR). Only conflicting medical decisions limit the far-reaching authority of nursing. According to the HÜR, the physician is no longer responsible for the assigned task. Before the nurse can perform the activity independently, the physician must make a diagnosis and indication and inform the nurse in a documented manner (§ 3 para. 1 HÜR). The physician remains responsible for ordering the transfer. However, the tort liability risk increases for the nurse, as the latter performs the delegated activity independently. This must be covered by private professional liability insurance or by adjusting the hospital's public liability insurance. The HÜR not only leads to a restructuring of the previous liability constellations, but also to a redistribution of costs. From an economic point of view, the reorganization of tasks results in savings in the area of personnel costs.

▶   The performance of port puncture by nurses is permissible according to the HÜR for intravenous applications of cytostatic drugs. Prerequisites are the nurse's "knowledge of indications, contraindications and complications of cytostatic drugs", the "mastery of basic skills for administering and monitoring infusion therapy" as well as "knowledge of port catheter care" (Annex HÜR, Part 2), which can be obtained within the framework of an additional qualification.

However, the application of the regulations requires that a model project in accordance with § 63 Para. 3 c SGB V is agreed between health insurance funds and service providers. Without a model project, the previous regulations apply. It remains to be seen whether the HÜR will prevail in practice.

Expert Standard Port Care

5

Barbara Fantl

Summary Since there are no uniform guidelines for the care of patients with central venous port systems in the Federal Republic of Germany to date, the recommendations formulated in the following chapter are based on guidelines of the Robert Koch Institute and on the many years of expertise of Universitätsklinikum Heidelberg (Heidelberg University Hospital). The standardized professional care of implanted port systems after port implantation is the most important measure to ensure permanent, complication-free and safe access for patients. A study conducted at Heidelberg University Hospital in which the reasons for port explantation were investigated in 385 patients clearly showed that port infection was the most frequent complication of implanted port systems and frequently led to explantation of the systems.

Since there is no uniform guideline for the care of patients with central venous port systems in the Federal Republic of Germany to date, the recommendations formulated in the following chapter are based on guidelines of the Robert Koch Institute and on the long-standing expertise of Heidelberg University Hospital.

The standardized professional care of implanted port systems is the most important measure after port implantation to ensure permanent, complication-free and safe access for patients.

A study at Heidelberg University Hospital (Fischer et al. 2008), which investigated the reasons for port explantation in 385 patients, clearly showed that port infection was the most frequent complication of implanted port systems and frequently led to explantation of the systems.

B. Fantl (✉)
Surgical Clinic and Clinic for Anaesthesiology, Heidelberg University Hospital, Heidelberg, Germany
e-mail: Barbara.Fantl@med.uni-heidelberg.de

© Springer-Verlag GmbH Germany, part of Springer Nature 2022
R. Hennes, G. Müller (eds.), *Port Care*,
https://doi.org/10.1007/978-3-662-64494-2_5

▶   Infections are the most common complication of implanted port
       systems and the most common cause of port explantation.

The handling of central venous ports is a medical activity that—like many
others—can be delegated to **trained** medical personnel.

If an employee—regardless of his or her training—feels unqualified or insuffi-
ciently qualified in the handling of central venous ports, he or she has a duty to refuse
this activity. Regardless of any delegation, the responsibility for implementation
always lies with the person performing the procedure (see also Chap. 4).

5.1   Care of Non-punctured Ports

For newly implanted ports, a change of dressing and wound inspection should be
performed on the second postoperative day.

The wound and wound environment should be examined for signs of infection
such as redness, swelling and pain. In case of abnormalities or wound healing
disorders, the implanting physician should be informed and, if possible, photo-
graphic documentation should be performed to monitor the progress. Due to a lack
of evidence regarding port flushing, there are different approaches. Some institutions
flush ports only after puncture, while others flush ports on a programmed basis every
6–8 weeks. Port system manufacturers recommend prophylactic flushing after
8–12 weeks. Since every puncture poses a potential risk of infection and no evidence
exists regarding the benefit of regular port flushing, no clear recommendation can
be made.

Two papers (Goossens et al. 2013, 2015; Bertoglio et al. 2012) addressing the
issue of blocking port systems demonstrated that routine blocking of port systems
with heparin solution does not result in an advantage over pure NaCl 0.9% solution.
There was never a significant difference in the laytime of the device; furthermore,
there was evidence of an increased risk of infection when using heparinized
solutions.

▶   No recommendation can be made for routine blocking with heparin.

5.2   Care of Punctured Ports

▶   **Practical tip** Do not puncture if there are local signs of infection such as
       redness, swelling and pain (Fig. 5.1).

Punctured ports with an inserted port cannula should have a dressing change every
48 h. The puncture site should be examined for signs of infection, hematoma and
secretion. If needles with a patch edge are used, a dressing change after 48 h does not
have to be performed. However, it must be ensured that the puncture site can be
inspected every 48 h in order to be able to act in case of changes.

Fig. 5.1 Infected port that should not be punctured under any circumstances. (Source: J. Rodrian, University Hospital Heidelberg)

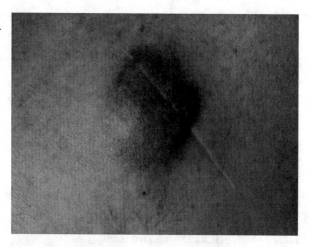

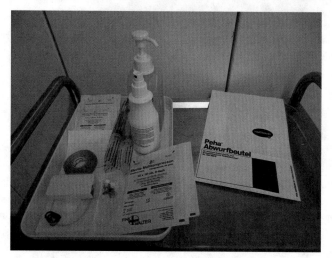

Fig. 5.2 Materials for puncturing a port. (Source: B. Fantl, Heidelberg University Hospital)

The needle itself is changed every 5–7 days. The companies recommend changing the needle after 7 days at the latest. After that, the manufacturing companies no longer accept responsibility for complications associated with port needles that remained for too long.

▶   **Practical tip** If the dressing becomes soiled or detached, change it immediately.

▶   Change cannula every 5–7 days.

Careful preparation is necessary for the puncture of a port. This includes the preparation of the material as well as that of the patient and his environment (Fig. 5.2).

5.2.1   Port Puncture Material

- Hand and skin disinfectants
- Non-sterile and sterile gloves
- Mouthguard
- Sterile compresses
- Two syringes of 10 ml NaCl 0.9% each
- Port cannula (appropriate size)
- Three-way stopcock with extension and sealing plug
- Disposal box
- Sterile pad

5.2.2   Material for the Dressing

- Single use slit compress 7.5 × 7.5 cm
- Single use compress 7.5 × 7.5 cm
- Adhesive bandages
- Band-aid

5.2.3   Patient Preparation

Since the puncture can be performed safely both in the sitting and lying position, the patient's wishes or needs can be sufficiently taken into account.

If the puncture is performed in a sitting position, the patient's back should be adequately stabilized to prevent backward evasive movements. If the patient does not perform the puncture independently, the head should be turned to the side facing away from the port.

5.3   Selection of the Port Cannula

Port chambers are designed for about 2000 punctures. Accordingly, they may only be punctured with special cannulas.

To prevent material from being punched out of the port membrane, the cannulas are specially ground. This displaces the membrane from the cannula during puncture and prevents silicone from being punched out.

The cannula diameter used should be adapted to the substances to be administered. For liquids with high viscosity, the cannula thickness should be at least 20 gauge.

▶ Only the special port cannulas intended for this purpose may be used for port puncture. Conventional cannulas can punch out material from the port membrane and thus damage the port.

According to the EU Directive on protection against needlestick injuries, only needles with a safety mechanism may be used since May 2013 (Directive 2010/32/EU, § 6(1)).

▶ **Practical tip** A suitable cannula size, but especially the cannula length, should be documented in the port passport or in the OP letter.

If the cannula length is not documented, the following criteria are used for selection:

- Depth of the port in the subcutaneous fat tissue
- Nutritional status of the patient

5.3.1   Complications with Inadequate Cannula Length (Fig. 5.3)

- Cannula's too long:
  - Cannula lies unstable in the stitch canal
  - Damage to the port membrane possible
  - The protrusion of the cannula above the level of the skin can cause the cannula to bend and break
- Too short a cannula:
  - Membrane is not punctured or only just punctured
  - Risk of extravasation with substance-dependent consequences such as tissue necrosis and inflammation (Fig. 5.4)

If, as in Fig. 5.3b, the safety mechanism of the port needle is triggered and then the port cannula is withdrawn, this also causes instability of the cannula. The membrane can be damaged in the process, and in the worst case the cannula can break off due to the instability.

▶ In case of puncture with the wrong cannula length, the cannula must be removed immediately and replaced by a suitable cannula.

5.4   Port Puncture

▶ **Practical tip** Port chamber systems are manufactured in different sizes, which can be felt during palpation. This results in different puncturing areas (Fig. 5.5).

After individual positioning of the patient, the upper body should be completely undressed and hygienic hand disinfection should have been performed. Subsequently, both the port chamber and its surroundings are palpated with non-sterile

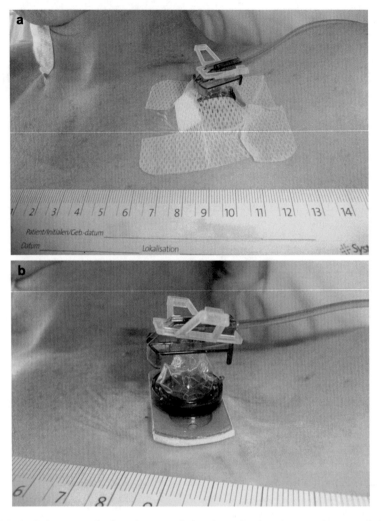

Fig. 5.3 (**a**, **b**) Incorrect selection of port needle length Duplication, the second port needle length must be deleted and of the dressing. (Source: J. Rodrian, University Hospital Heidelberg)

gloves. The skin surrounding the port chamber should be examined for signs of infection and the patient should be asked about pain in the port area.

▶ If the patient reports discomfort in the area of the port pocket, the planned puncture must be aborted and a physician informed.

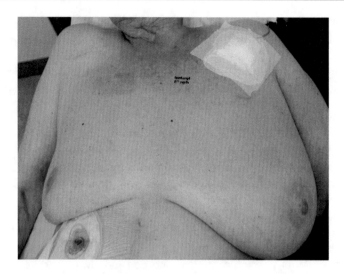

Fig. 5.4 Extravasation of 1500 ml of parenteral nutrition due to port cannula chosen too short. (Source: J. Rodrian, University Hospital Heidelberg)

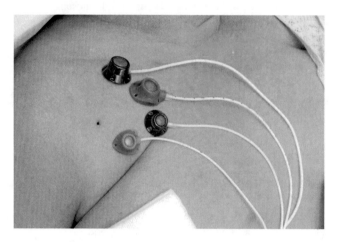

Fig. 5.5 Different port chamber size duplication. (Source: J. Rodrian, University Hospital Heidelberg)

▶   Redness, swelling, and tenderness may indicate both infection and systemic leakage.

After palpation and assessment, disinfection of the puncture site is started according to the RKI guideline (recommendation category 1B). While the puncture site is drying, the non-sterile gloves are disposed of, a new hygienic hand disinfection is performed and the materials for the port puncture are prepared sterilely. It is also advisable to put on non-sterile gloves for this purpose.

Then, after renewed hygienic hand disinfection, the sterile gloves are put on, the port cannula and the three-way stopcock are sterilely vented and the clamp on the cannula tube is closed (if a clamp is available). The port chamber is now palpated with one hand and securely fixed with two fingers (Fig. 5.6a, with the other hand the cannula is inserted vertically into the port chamber (Fig. 5.6b). After the puncture, the clamp is opened to check the position and blood is aspirated. If no blood can be aspirated, an attempt is made to flush the port with increased caution.

▶ Injection must be possible at any time without resistance!

If the port cannot be flushed without resistance, the cannula must be removed and a new puncture attempt shall be made with a new port cannula. If the port is used for continuous infusion therapy, the port needle should be changed every 5–7 days.

▶ **Practical tip** The initial puncture of a port is the responsibility of an experienced physician. Since each port is punctured intraoperatively by the surgeon for position control, a lying port has always had its initial puncture. Thus, any trained medical professional may puncture such a port.

For decannulation of the port, the same hygienic guidelines apply as for puncture. The port is flushed with 10 ml NaCl 0.9% and blocked. The port chamber is then stabilized with two fingers, the port needle is removed vertically from the port housing and safely discarded. The puncture site is disinfected and then a sterile plaster is applied, which can usually be removed after 24 h without replacement.

▶ To avoid the formation of a puncture channel, each new puncture should be made at a different puncture site (Fig. 5.7).

5.5 Blood Sampling from the Port

To prevent possible port occlusion due to improper flushing, blood should not be drawn through the port if peripheral venous status is good.

If peripheral blood sampling is not possible, the port can be used. In this case, a port cannula with a minimum diameter of 20 gauge is indispensable. After blood collection, the port should be flushed with at least 30 ml NaCl 0.9%. To ensure that all blood cells have been flushed from the port, 50 ml NaCl 0.9% is optimal. The port must be flushed using the push-and-go technique to ensure that all blood particles are flushed out of the chamber (Fig. 5.8).

Only syringes with a capacity of at least 10 ml may be used to flush the port. Smaller syringes can develop such high pressure that the silicone membrane can be blown off (Fig. 5.9). This has catastrophic consequences for the patient. The port must be explanted or replaced.

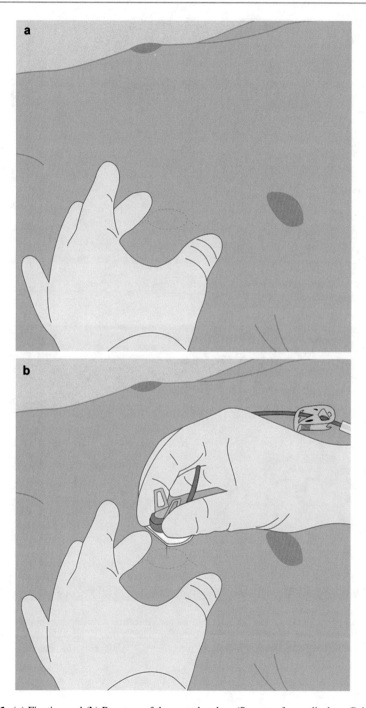

Fig. 5.6 (**a**) Fixation and (**b**) Puncture of the port chamber. (Source: pfm medical ag, Cologne)

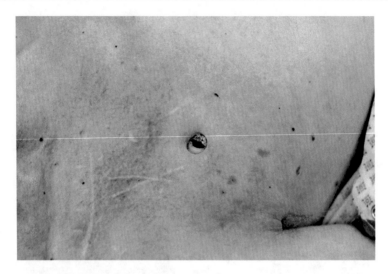

Fig. 5.7 Wound healing disorder duplication after formation of a stitch canal. (Source: J. Rodrian, University Hospital Heidelberg)

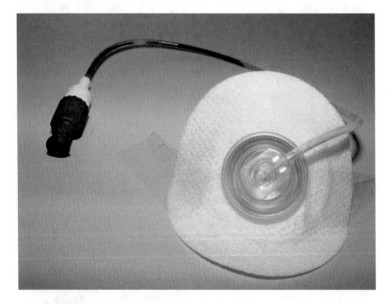

Fig. 5.8 Blood coagulation in the port needle tube due to insufficient rinsing after blood collection. Patient came from home care. Here, the port was not sufficiently flushed after blood sampling, was occluded and had to be explanted. (Source: S. Eismann, NCT, University Hospital Heidelberg)

Fig. 5.9 Bulging of the silicone membrane from the port chamber due to the use of a 2 ml syringe with unauthorized pressure. (From Ports, Springer Hennes and Hofmann 2016)

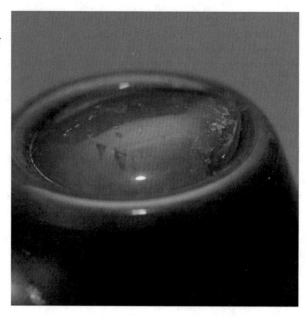

► **Practical tip** When flushing the catheter, flush at an uneven pace, the so-called push-and-go technique. This will remove more debris from the catheter wall than flushing at a steady pace or using a continuous infusion.

5.6   Procedure for Port Infection

If there are clinical indications of a port infection, the infusion therapy must be stopped immediately. Blood cultures should be taken from both the port and a peripheral vein for further diagnostic confirmation and targeted antibiotic therapy. One way to sanitize a port catheter system is to administer a 3-ml block of taurolidine for 48–72 h. After this time, the taurolidine is removed from the port by aspiration and blood cultures are taken again from both the port and peripherally. If possible, injection into the patient should be avoided, as bacteria may have accumulated in the taurolidine solution in the event of a catheter infection and then be flushed into the patient. This can lead to an allergic reaction, such as chills and fever.

Depending on the clinical condition, laboratory and signs of infection, the further procedure must be evaluated. In case of persistent infection, explantation of the port system must be considered.

▶ **Practical tip** Taurolidine is not an antibiotic. It is bactericidal and effective against all tested germs (approx. 500) including MRSA and VRE.

In order to reduce the risk of infection in immunosuppressed patients, it has proven effective to prophylactically provide the port with a permanent taurolidine block according to the recommendation from the care guidelines for ports of Heidelberg University Hospital, which, however, must be replaced after 30 days. The stability of taurolidine is no longer guaranteed after 30 days. This is also recommended for patients who have had a port infection. If the solution is applied to the patient when the taurolidine block is changed, this is not a problem because the solution was blocked when the patient was free of infection.

▶ **Practical tip** Taurolidine is a derivative of amino acids. The watery solution has a bactericidal effect and is converted to the amino acid taurine in the bloodstream. Taurolidine as a permanent catheter block solution can reduce the deposition of a biofilm on the catheter wall.

5.7 Documentation

All procedures performed on the port should be recorded promptly and completely in the patient's chart. After each puncture, the cannula size, the appearance of the port environment and the change of dressing must be documented.

If there is evidence of infection, that fact and the action taken must also be recorded.

5.8 Patient and Family Education

Port infections are predominantly due to poor hygiene in handling the systems. Since puncture and infusion therapy in the home environment is increasingly being carried out by patients themselves or by their relatives, great importance should be posed on their detailed and comprehensible training (Fig. 5.10). Training measures can already begin before implantation and should include the following points:

- Only trained personnel may puncture and use the port.
- The patient shares responsibility for his or her port and should encourage doctors and nurses to comply with applicable hygiene guidelines.
- The port passport should be carried at all times.
- In general, care should be taken to maintain a clean environment.
- Hygiene guidelines must always be followed.
- Use of disinfectant, non-sterile/sterile gloves and sterile compresses.

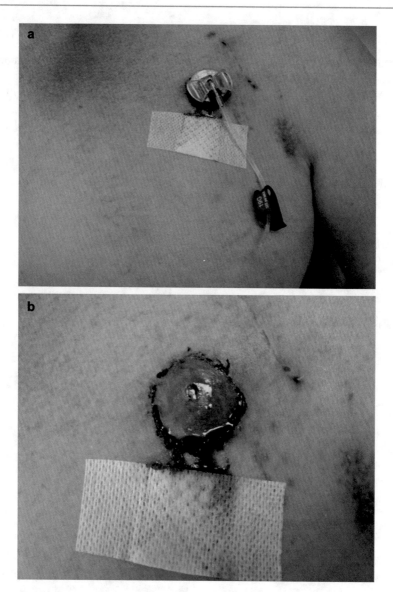

Fig. 5.10 (**a**, **b**) Patient came from home care. The social care unit had cut the port needle tube because the caring nurse had not dared to pull the needle. The port was infected. (Source: S. Eismann, NCT, University Hospital Heidelberg)

5.9   Conclusion

Port systems can be used for many years. For this purpose, it is imperative that only uniformly and optimally trained personnel perform punctures, infusions, injections and blood sampling at the port. Uniform standards of care and regular training in the various facilities must be required.

The proper staff, patient and family education helps reduce and prevent port infections.

References

Bertoglio S et al (2012) Efficacy of normal saline versus heparinized saline solution for locking catheters of totally implantable long-term central vascular access devices in adult cancer patients. Cancer Nurs 35(4):E35–E42

Fischer L et al (2008) Reasons for explantation of totally implantable access ports: a multivariate analysis of 385 consecutive patients. Ann Surg Oncol 15(4):1124–1129

Goossens GA, De WY, Jerome M, Fieuws S, Janssens C, Stas M et al (2015) Diagnostic accuracy of the catheter injection and aspiration (CINAS) classification for assessing the function of totally implantable venous access devices. Support Care Cancer 24(2):755–761

Goossens GA et al (2013 Jul) Comparing normal saline versus diluted heparin to lock non-valved totally implantable venous access devices in cancer patients: a randomised, non-inferiority, open trial. Ann Oncol 24(7):1892–1899

Hennes R, Hofmann HAF (2016) Ports. Springer, Heidelberg. ISBN 978-3-662-436440-0

Wound Care and Dressing Changes

6

Barbara Fantl

Summary Wound care and dressing—just like the puncture—must be carried out according to hygienic guidelines. The dressing should always be applied under sterile conditions. This chapter explains the principles of wound care and dressing changes.

Wound care and dressing—just like the puncture—must be carried out according to hygienic guidelines.

▶ The dressing should always be applied under sterile conditions.

6.1 Port Needles

The variety on the port needle product market is now very large. It is advisable for a medical facility to commit to one product if possible, in order to create a unity that ensures standardized training in the safe handling of port needles for staff. This guarantees a higher level of safety than if different products with different handling are in circulation.

It is important that only safety port pins are being used (Figs. 6.1, 6.2 and 6.3).

▶ According to the EU Directive on protection against needlestick injuries, only needles with a safety mechanism may be used since May 2013 (Directive 2010/32/EU, § 6 para. 1).

Only suitable port needles may be used to puncture a port.

Port needles have a special cut that prevents the membrane from being punched out when piercing the port membrane (Fig. 6.4).

B. Fantl (✉)
Surgical Clinic and Clinic for Anaesthesiology, Heidelberg University Hospital, Heidelberg, Germany
e-mail: Barbara.Fantl@med.uni-heidelberg.de

© Springer-Verlag GmbH Germany, part of Springer Nature 2022
R. Hennes, G. Müller (eds.), *Port Care*,
https://doi.org/10.1007/978-3-662-64494-2_6

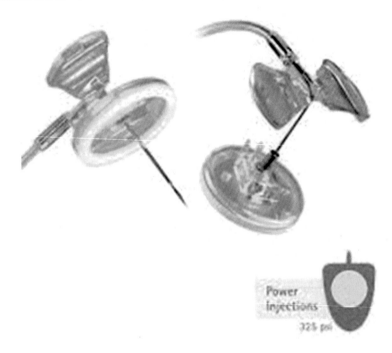

Fig. 6.1 Safety pin from the Braun company

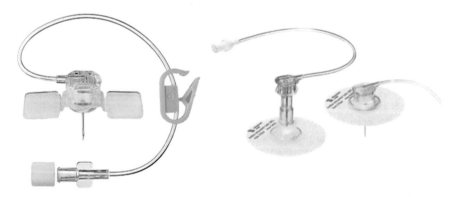

Fig. 6.2 Fresenius safety pin

The port needle lengths should be selected depending on the patient's constitution (Fig. 6.5). Needle lengths vary between 10 and 38 mm. The lumen of the port needles is given in gauge. If one wishes to draw blood through the port and administer infusions with higher viscosity, a port needle with at least 20 gauge must be selected. Needles with a smaller lumen would occlude due to the higher viscosity.

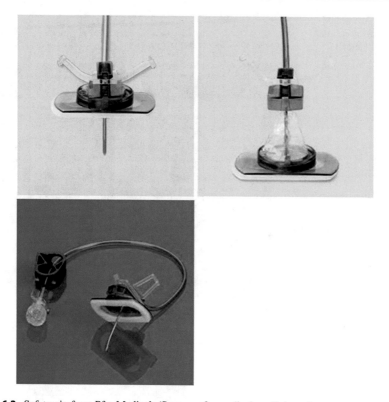

Fig. 6.3 Safety pin from Pfm Medical. (Source: pfm medical ag, Cologne)

▶ **Practical tip** The gauge unit is the unit of measurement for the outer diameter of cannulas. It is inversely related to the diameter. This means that the smaller the gauge unit, the larger the diameter of the cannula.

6.2   Bandage

Unfortunately, there is no standard port dressing on the market as of today. In any case, the bandage must be applied and fixed in such a way that slipping of the needle during movement is avoided (Fig. 6.6).

Fig. 6.4 Port needle grinding/trocar needle (PacuMed GmbH)

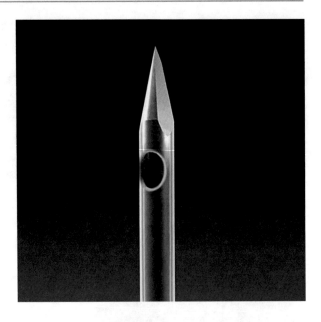

Fig. 6.5 Incorrectly selected port needle: The needle is too long. (Source: Rudolph University Hospital Heidelberg)

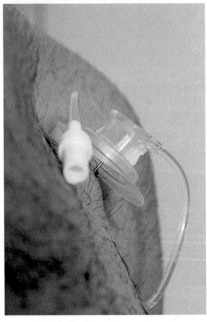

Fig. 6.6 Port needle
dressing. (Source: Rudolph
University Hospital
Heidelberg)

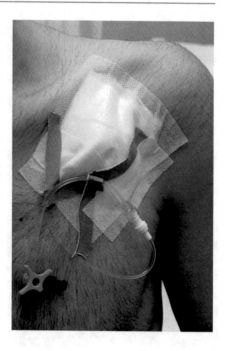

▶   **Practical tip** The dressing must be fixed in such a way that the needle
cannot slip during movement.

6.2.1   Dressing Materials for Needles without Plaster

- Single use slit compress 7.5 × 7.5 cm
- Single use compress 7.5 × 7.5 cm
- Fixation bandage/foil
- Band-aid strips

▶   When applying the dressing, care must be taken to ensure that the slit
dressing is **not** pushed under the cover plate/wing, but is applied over
it. This prevents the needle from lifting off.

6.2.2   Dressing Materials for Needles with Plaster

- Wide self-adhesive fixation bandage approx. 10 × 10 cm or
- Foil dressing approx. 10 × 10 cm

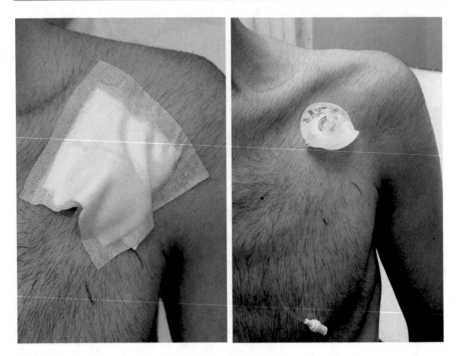

Fig. 6.7 Detached port needle dressing. (Source: Rudolph University Hospital Heidelberg)

When applying the dressing, a wound inspection for signs of infection, hematoma and secretion must of course be carried out beforehand.

The dressing should be changed every 48 h to allow the puncture site to be assessed. In the case of port needles with plaster, the plaster fixation should be removed after 48 h so that the puncture site can be assessed from the outside. The plaster of the needle does not have to be removed for this purpose.

▶   **Practical tip** If the dressing becomes soiled or detached, change the dressing immediately (Fig. 6.7).

6.3   Connections

All port needles that have **a** clamp on the tube do **not** have **an** integrated check valve at the connection point. Therefore, the clamp must be closed before any manipulation to avoid backflow of blood or aspiration of air.

All port needles that **do not have a** clamp are equipped with an integrated non-return valve. However, these must still be closed at the connection point with a sterile cap to prevent the intrusion of germs.

6.4   Puncture and Connection

A port catheter can be punctured up to approx. 2000 times. This results in a lying time of several years. To avoid the formation of a puncture channel with a punching defect, a different puncture site must always be selected when changing the needle.

▶   **Practical tip** The skin over the port chamber can be moved. Therefore, even with small port chamber systems, you can always choose a different puncture site.

Any manipulation of the port system must be performed under sterile conditions. To connect an infusion to the port system, hygienic hand disinfection should be performed before placing a sterile compress underneath, spraying and removing the cap. Disinfectant is then sprayed into the cone, and after 15 s exposure time, the residues of the disinfectant are tapped out of the device (https://www.rki.de/DE/Content/Infekt/Krankenhaushygiene/Kommission/Downloads/Gefaesskat_Rili.pdf?__blob=publicationFile). This serves to prevent infection and is a new guideline of the RKI (https://www.rki.de/DE/Content/Infekt/Krankenhaushygiene/Kommission/Downloads/Gefaesskat_Rili.pdf?__blob=publicationFile).

6.5   Handling Water

When the port needle is in place, showering should be avoided if possible. Even with so-called waterproof plasters, water can enter the dressing through microfolds that are not visible to the naked eye. This creates a moist chamber which is an ideal breeding ground for germs.

Therefore, the patient is advised to shower only underneath the lying port needle and to take care that no splashing water gets on the dressing.

When changing the needle, the patient can be offered to take a shower between the removal of the needle and the new insertion. A sterile plaster should be applied to the puncture site and a foil dressing should also be applied, which should be removed immediately after the shower.

This is often problematic in home use, as domestic care services often come to the patients to change the needle and there is usually no time for showering between pulling and inserting the needle. In this case, the patient should be precisely informed about the dangers of showering with the needle in the lying position. If a shower is nevertheless taken with the needle in place, a new dressing must be applied immediately after the shower. Care must be taken to ensure that the skin is disinfected intensively and that the exposure time is observed.

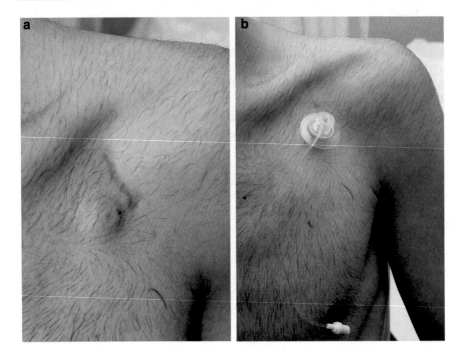

Fig. 6.8 (**a, b**) Hairy puncture site. (Source: Rudolph University Hospital Heidelberg)

▶ When the port needle is in place, water should generally not come into contact with the dressing and the needle, as there is an increased risk of bacterial colonization at the puncture site. A bacterial colonization can lead to a port infection.

6.6   Handling Hair in the Puncture Area

In general, care should be taken to ensure that the puncture area is free of hair, as hair is always a source of germs. Therefore, the puncture site should be shaved before puncturing the port (Fig. 6.8).

Further Reading

EU-Richtlinie 2010/32/EU. www.nadelstichverletzung.de/eu-richtlinie.html
Pflegeleitlinie Universitätsklinikum Heidelberg. www.klinikum.uni-heidelberg.de/
    Pflegeleitlinien.133798.0.html?&L=1

Intraoperative and Postoperative Care of Port Patients

7

Birgit Appelhoff and Lisa Moser

Summary Structured and well-organized management of responsible care is an important component of a successful course of treatment for a port patient. This chapter provides information on the crucial nursing measures.

7.1   General

A structured and well-organized management of responsible care is an important component of a successful course of treatment for a port patient. The nursing measures are crucial here.

The organization of surgical treatment begins on the day of surgery with the patient's admission via a day-care hospital/an outpatient monitoring area with seamless care from admission to discharge with the discharge interview from the medical and nursing side.

The implantation of a port can be performed under general or local anesthesia. Another possibility is the combination of analgosedation in combination with a local anesthesia procedure.

B. Appelhoff (✉) · L. Moser
Surgical Clinic and Clinic for Anaesthesiology, Heidelberg University Hospital, Heidelberg, Germany
e-mail: Birgit.Appelhoff@med.uni-heidelberg.de; Lisa.Moser@med.uni-heidelberg.de

© Springer-Verlag GmbH Germany, part of Springer Nature 2022
R. Hennes, G. Müller (eds.), *Port Care*,
https://doi.org/10.1007/978-3-662-64494-2_7

▶ **Practical tip** Patients do not need to be fasting for port implantation if the operation is performed under local anaesthesia. It is then even advantageous if the patients have had breakfast, as experience has shown that they are more relaxed and calmer and complain less about nausea.

7.1.1 Reasons for Port Implantation under Intubation Anesthesia

- Intolerances/allergic reactions to local anaesthetics
- Anxiety/phobias
- Implantation within another surgical treatment under general anesthesia
- Personal urgent reasons of the patient
- Mentally disabled patients and children

7.2 Intraoperative Care

In the case of port implantation under local anaesthesia, the patient requires empathic care during the procedure. This requires the operating room staff to communicate in a way that gives the patient security and confidence.

In some hospitals, it is possible to let the patient listen to music or use his headphones in the operating room if he is very agitated.

▶ **Practical tip** Especially in the case of longer procedures and difficulties during implantation, the surgical team should remain calm towards the patient and radiate competence.

If it is necessary to use the port immediately on the day of implantation, the surgeon may insert a port needle intraoperatively...the surgeon may leave the port needle in place, after the initial puncture.

▶ The initial puncture is always the responsibility of an experienced physician. The intraoperative port puncture is considered the initial puncture (Fig. 5.2).

7.2.1 Intraoperative Problems and Complications

Since various intraoperative problems and complications may occur, constant monitoring of the patient is required. In particular, attention should be paid to the following complications:

- Cardiac arrhythmia → Port catheter tip is too deep in the right atrium/ventricle
- Difficulty in advancing the catheter may result in the need for vascular imaging with X-ray contrast medium. In this case, the renal function/values must be taken into account to determine the extent to which the administration of contrast medium is possible at all.
- Acute restlessness and anxiety states

7.3 Postoperative Care

If the procedure is performed as part of outpatient surgery, the patient can be discharged after a doctor's visit and checking of vital signs if the intraoperative and postoperative course is uncomplicated. After the port implantation, the patient's vital signs are checked and the special port documents (port passport, OP letter, the documents of the port manufacturer) are handed out to the patient. At the Heidelberg Port Center, all patients also receive a port brochure (Fig. 7.1) to inform patients and relatives. If no intraoperative or postoperative complications have occurred, the patient can leave the clinic after a detailed consultation.

7.3.1 Information of the Consultation

- Suture material used (absorbable/non-absorbable)
- Physical rest for approx. 2 weeks. During this time, the patient should not perform any heavy physical work, should not work overhead and should avoid sports such as tennis, swimming and martial arts as well as heavy lifting in order to support undisturbed wound healing
- Showering is possible from the first postoperative day onwards
- Bathing is recommended only after wound healing is complete
- Dealing with painkillers
- Information about signs of infection such as redness, overheating, suddenly increasing or newly occurring pain in the area of the surgical wound
- Carrying the passport for all radiological examinations (especially CT and MRT diagnostics)

> **Practical tip** The local anaesthetic is effective for between 1 and 6 hours, depending on the choice of local anaesthetic. As pain may still occur after the local anaesthetic has finished working, the patient is discharged with a pain prescription (a suitable analgesic is prescribed for the patient).

In case of any changes or uncertainties regarding the port, e.g., a permanent foreign body sensation, the patient is recommended to return quickly.

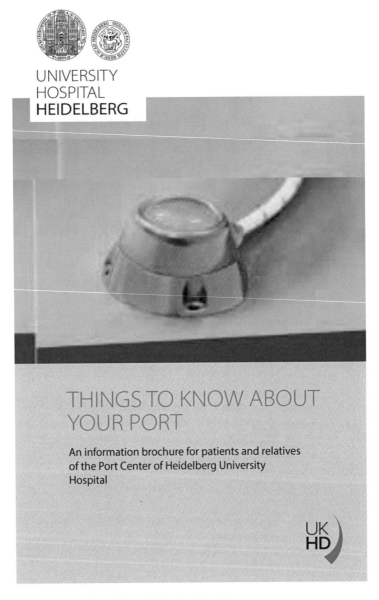

Fig. 7.1 Port brochure of Heidelberg University Hospital

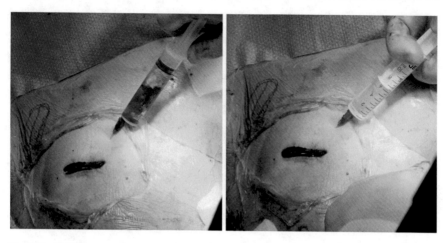

Fig. 7.2 (**a**, **b**) Intraoperative functional test (Source: Rudolph, University Hospital Heidelberg)

7.4 The First Puncture

The first check for functionality of the port system is always performed intraoperatively by the physician to be implanted who performs the implantation (Fig. 7.2).

Palpation of the port chamber is performed with 2–3 fingers of one hand (Fig. 5.6a).

▶ **Practical tip** The appropriate needle length is selected on the basis of the extent of the subcutis present. As the intraoperative administration of the local anaesthetic may cause swelling of the tissue over the port chamber or the implantation may sometimes cause hematomas in the surgical area, it is possible that the needle length will have to be adjusted after wound healing has been completed.

7.5 Conclusion

The empathic and responsible monitoring and nursing care of the patient intra- and postoperatively is an essential component of competent treatment of a port patient. Ensuring patient safety and minimizing risks and complications are paramount in this regard.

Special Features of Port Care for Oncological Patients

8

Susann Eismann

Summary Oncology is the main field for application of port systems. Due to the severity of their disease, many patients are dependent on a permanently safe vascular access.

While Hickmann catheters are often used in pediatric oncology because of the "puncture trauma", a port is almost always chosen for adults. Many patients have a poor venous status, which eliminates peripheral intravenous catheters as a permanent solution. It is important to educate patients about port systems early in therapy. The nurse plays an important role here, as he or she can sensitively advise the oncological patients about the advantages of a port system after the necessary cytostatic therapy and port systems have been explained in the doctor's consultation.

8.1 The Right Access for Cytostatic Therapy

The choice of the optimal vascular access depends on the duration and type of the planned therapy. The application of vasotoxic substances (e.g. anthracyclines) or cytostatic continuous infusions (e.g. via elastomer pumps) should only be carried out via safe central access points. This minimizes the risk of extravasation.

In the case of poor venous conditions or a high probability of additional parenteral nutrition during the course of the disease, it is important to implant a port catheter system early on in order to avoid unnecessarily traumatizing patients with unsuccessful venipunctures.

When oncological patients are treated with a port system in the day-clinical/outpatient area, unnecessary hospital stays can be prevented, since outpatient care with parenteral nutrition or even pure fluid substitution can be quickly organized for the domestic sector.

S. Eismann (✉)
National Center for Tumor Diseases (NCT) Heidelberg, Heidelberg University Hospital, Heidelberg, Germany
e-mail: susann.eismann@med.uni-heidelberg.de

© Springer-Verlag GmbH Germany, part of Springer Nature 2022
R. Hennes, G. Müller (eds.), *Port Care*,
https://doi.org/10.1007/978-3-662-64494-2_8

8.1.1   Position Control of the Port Needle

After aseptically placing the port needle, it is important to check its position. Some port systems always have back flow (blood can be aspirated), but some never aspirate blood. With some port systems, blood can be aspirated after a puncture and then not again. The cause is often hypotension (e.g. due to general weakness, severe weight loss), insufficient fluid intake by the patient (e.g. in cases of extreme diarrhoea, tumour cachexia, ascites) or the altered position of the port catheter tip on the wall of the superior vena cava or in an ostium of the vein wall.

If a port system is not showing any back flow, it is still important to ensure that the port needle is positioned correctly. Even if the bottom is felt when the port needle is inserted, a lack of aspiration of blood can confuse both patient and caregiver. A volume of 20–100 ml NaCl 0.9% can be infused briskly for positional testing. The application must be feasible without resistance and must not cause the patient any pain. Meanwhile, the port environment must be observed intensively. If there is no swelling, the patient is not in pain and the puncture site does not turn wet, then the port needle is in the correct position and therapy can be started.

▶   **Practical Tip**
     Port needles that are positioned correctly but feel very sluggish can make therapy difficult or impossible. It is important here that a port thrombosis and dislocation of the port catheter tube/leakage can be ruled out by a vein duplex ultrasound or fluoroscopy.

Very rarely, a port catheter tube can completely kink or dislocate in the patient. This is often caused by extreme sports activities (e.g. judo or squash). A tingling sensation in the neck area of the patient when flushing the port system can sometimes indicate a dislocation of the catheter tube and requires surgical correction.

In obese patients it is possible that the port lies very deep in the subcutaneous tissue, which makes the puncture even more difficult. In these very overweight patients, the port may tilt or even completely rotate, making puncture difficult or impossible. Surgical correction is often required. A correctly punctured deep port must be fixed particularly well and, if necessary, checked more often during therapy. Especially in obese patients a dislocation of the port needle from the silicone membrane can occur, as the subcutis presses against the attachment plate of the port needle and dislocates it from the septum. Port puncture in obese patients is often easier with the patient lying down. A cushion in the thoracic region allows an optimized V-positioning and the port is easier to puncture.

8.1.2   Fixation of the Port Needle for Cytostatic Therapy

The use of a port needle with integrated plaster is optimal to reduce extravasation. An additional covering with adhesive bandage or a foil bandage increases the adhesive surface. It is advisable to fix the port needle tube in place. The dressing must be changed as quickly as possible if it becomes soiled or soaked, and the position of the port needle must be checked. Many patients have the port needle additionally padded with sterile compresses under the adhesive dressing or foil dressing in the day-clinic/outpatient area.

If port needles are used without an integrated plaster, sterile covering and, depending on the patient's activity, reinforced securing is essential. Sterile clip plasters, for example, can be helpful here.

▶ **Practical tip** Using the optimal port needle length for the patient is essential and prevents extravasation. A needle that is too short often makes it impossible to flush the port and must be adjusted. A needle that is too long can break off or slip out more quickly.

8.2 Complications of Cytostatic Therapy Via a Port

The correct use of a port catheter system for cytostatic therapy does not prevent extravasation. Careful inspection of the port needle by the nursing staff before and during therapy is essential. In addition, the patient must also be aware and report any pain, swelling or oozing bandage immediately. If extravasation is suspected, therapy must be stopped immediately and the port needle tested. If extravasation occurs, a physician should be consulted so that the substance-specific measures can be taken immediately (Figs. 8.1, 8.2, and 8.3).

▶ It is important not to remove the port needle immediately in order to remove any extravasation of the cytostatic drug through the port needle.

8.3 Drip Speed and Cytostatic Therapy with Elastomer Pumps

In recent years, almost only high-pressure ports have been implanted in Germany. These ports can be run at 5 ml/s. If several infusions are running simultaneously, an adjustment to the maximum total drip rate is important.

Frequently, in the day-care clinic/outpatient setting, medications are also infused via infusions using an elastomer pump after cytostatic therapy. This makes it possible to administer drugs that have to run for several days in the home environment. For this, the patient must be well trained in the use of his therapy pump and good fixation of the needle is essential. Most commonly, 5-fluorouracil (5FU) is administered in these pumps with run times of 1–7 days. Therapy with elastomer pumps in the home setting is only possible via central access, whereby a port catheter system is to be favoured. The pump connection should always be fixed with adhesive bandage or dressing foil. After completion of cytostatic therapy, regardless of whether via infusion or elastomer pump, the port should first be rinsed with carrier

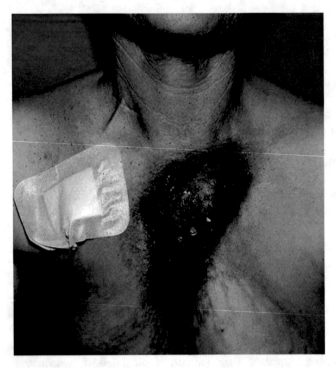

Fig. 8.1 Extravasation due to doxorubicin. (Source: S. Eismann, NCT, University Hospital Heidelberg)

solution. Finally, before removing the port needle, the port system must be flushed quickly with 30 ml NaCl 0.9% using the push-and-go technique.

The running speed of an elastomer pump varies somewhat depending on the patient's activity, body temperature and ambient temperature. A sluggish port catheter system can also influence the running time and extend it unnecessarily. Therefore, it is important that the cause (needle too short, needle too thin, port thrombosis, kinked port catheter, etc.) be identified and the problem be corrected. Documentation of the maximum possible runtime is useful as a follow-up.

When using elastomer pumps for therapy, the port needle may "work its way out" of the port in active, obese or restlessly sleeping patients with no fluid passing through anymore. The needle then no longer lies optimally in the port chamber, but is partially stuck in the port membrane with the needle tip. By applying light pressure with the flat hand on the port needle, the position can often be corrected without having to change the needle. If this is not successful, the port must be tested for proper functioning by flushing the port needle with NaCl 0.9% and changing the needle.

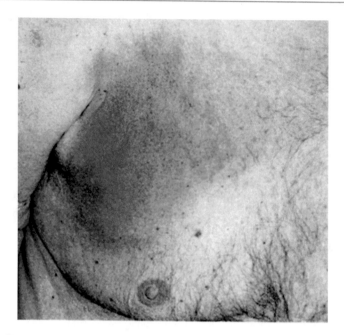

Fig. 8.2 Port extravasation oxaliplatin. (Source: S. Eismann, NCT, University Hospital Heidelberg)

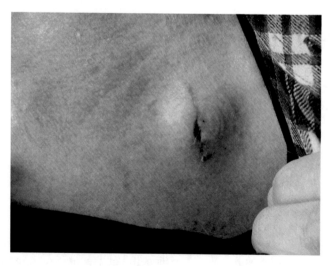

Fig. 8.3 Wound healing disorder under chemotherapy. Port was implanted 1 week before. (Source: S. Eismann, NCT, University Hospital Heidelberg)

▶ To be sure of the type of port system implanted, it is important for the patient to carry the port identification card with him/her at all times. The manufacturer's important recommendations for use are noted in it.

8.4 Special Features of Arm Ports and Groin Ports

Arm ports are now implanted only very rarely because of the increased risk of thrombosis due to the long catheter tube. These ports are implanted near the crook of the arm. In addition, they restrict arm flexion and can also cause pressure damage to nerves and vessels of the arm.

In patients with extensive thrombosis in the thoracic region, sometimes only the implantation of an inguinal port is possible. If the port chamber of the inguinal port is placed on the tensor fascia latae muscle—on the outer side of the thigh, proximally—it can be punctured very easily and does not show an increased incidence of infection. The patient should be positioned comfortably during the puncture and should not be mobilized during the infusion. Good intimate hygiene of the patient reduces infections. After infusions via an arm or groin port, it is recommended to rinse with at least 20 ml NaCl 0.9% using the push-and-go technique.

8.5 Parenteral Nutrition Via a Port

Patients who are fed parenterally have special requirements for the port catheter system. Here, too, compliance with hygiene guidelines and strict aseptic procedures are essential. The port needle must have as large an inner diameter as possible (19 or 20 G), since the high-caloric nutrient mixtures are viscous and can clog the port. Immediately after parenteral nutrition, the port must always be quickly rinsed with at least 20 ml NaCl 0.9%. It is even better to use 30 ml NaCl 0.9% in push-and-go technique.

The port needle must be changed every 5–7 days. When changing the needle, the puncture site must always be varied to prevent necrosis, pressure points and punch defects at the puncture site.

Daily inspection of the insertion site and checking the position of the port needle before parenteral nutrition can reduce port infections and prevent extravasation from high-calorie nutritional solutions.

▶ Many different professional groups work with port systems. Not all users are always familiar with aseptic handling. It is all the more relevant that the patient also knows key steps in handling his or her port system and that the importance of disinfection and needle change is pointed out again and again. The training of patients and relatives is becoming increasingly crucial here.

Port Supply in Outpatient Care

9

Halka Nehring and Anna Mindrup

Summary Not only in the inpatient setting, but also in the outpatient setting, the port as a vascular access that is available at any time and can often be punctured represents the basis for therapy with hyperosmolar infusions, as embodied by parenteral nutrition and cytostatic infusions. This enables patients to receive or continue their required therapy in their familiar environment. This is often accompanied by a better therapy outcome and a gain in quality of life. In order to make this possible, a well-networked cooperation of the professional groups involved in the care is required. A close-knit information and communication network is indispensable, in which the patient and his relatives are also integrated (Fig. 9.1).

9.1 Areas of Responsibility

9.1.1 Doctor

According to the resolution of the Federal Joint Committee of Germany (G-BA) of December 17, 2015, hospital physicians can prescribe home nursing care for up to 7 calendar days after discharge in the same way as contract physicians (G-BA 2015b). Furthermore, the forwarding of information on prescriptions made to the contract physician who continues treatment is regulated in order to ensure "seamless follow-up care" (G-BA 2015a). This was intended to close a gap in care that had repeatedly occurred up to this point, e.g. on weekends and public holidays. However, discharge prescriptions, which enable the immediate provision of medicines

H. Nehring (✉)
Peine, Germany

A. Mindrup
Hohenzollern Pharmacy, Sterile Manufacturing & Homecare, Münster, Germany
e-mail: a.mindrup@hza.de

© Springer-Verlag GmbH Germany, part of Springer Nature 2022
R. Hennes, G. Müller (eds.), *Port Care*,
https://doi.org/10.1007/978-3-662-64494-2_9

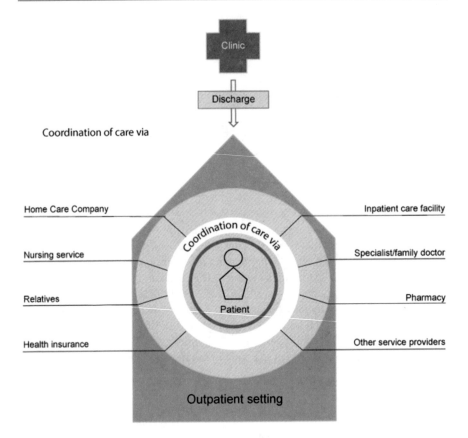

Fig. 9.1 Communication and action partners in outpatient care

and medical aids for 7 calendar days, and thus provide seamless continuous care at any time, are only slowly being introduced here.

The contracting outpatient physician in the practice or medical care centre (MVZ) prescribes further home care within the framework of outpatient care on the basis of the "G-BA guideline on the prescription of home care (Home Care Guideline)" (G-BA 2015b). The scope of the measures and the prescribability depend on the individual needs of the patient and the list of services. The prescription is made on the form "Home health care prescription"; the relevant diagnoses, the services to be provided as well as the start, frequency and duration of the measures must be stated.

The hospital or contract physician determines the respective treatment regime and provides this in writing to the provider and the nursing service. The contract physician also prescribes the medicines, remedies and aids required for the therapy before the outpatient treatment begins. The transferability of medical activities to registered nurses (e.g. port puncture) is regulated in the "Transfer Guideline of the G-BA" of 21 March 2012 (G-BA 2012); it is patient-related and also requires the written form. In the course of treatment, all changes in therapy must be documented in writing.

In the case of abnormalities, problems and uncertainties, prompt consultation with the doctor and information of the other people involved in the care is essential for an optimal treatment process and success.

9.1.2 Case Management/Discharge Management/Transition Management

The seamless transition from inpatient to outpatient care requires the earliest possible and most careful planning, coordination and supervision. Since 2007, patients have had a statutory right "for care management, in particular to solve problems during the transition to the various care areas"; this also includes specialist follow-up care. The service providers concerned ensure that the insured person receives appropriate follow-up care and provide each other with the necessary information. They are to be supported by the health insurance funds in fulfilling this task", regulated in § 11 (4) SGB V in the "Act to Strengthen Competition in Statutory Health Insurance" (SGB V 2020). "Care management and any transmission of data required for this purpose may only take place with the consent and after prior information of the insured person" (SGB V 2020).

In many hospitals, professional teams, mostly consisting of nursing staff and/or social services, have been established in recent years. However, there is no uniform procedure for interface management. Patients can be registered both via the ward and via the social services or discharge management. The selection of service providers can be direct (service provider and nursing service are requested by the hospital after consultation and with the patient's consent) or indirect (an involved nursing service recommends a service provider from its existing network partners after consultation and with the patient's consent, or vice versa).

The outpatient prescribing physician should already be informed about the planned treatment measures during the patient's inpatient stay.

9.1.3 Homecare Companies/Service Providers

Outpatient providers, also known as homecare companies, have their field of activity in the complex and specialized care and support of patients in the domestic environment. They work in close cooperation with doctors, nursing services, health insurance companies and one or more cooperating pharmacies. There are various structures within the homecare company. Within the complex care situation, the employees of the field service fulfil the tasks of a care manager as a central element: they communicate with the professional groups involved, the patients and their relatives and, if necessary, ensure the smooth transition from inpatient to outpatient care as an external interface. In order to create an optimal care situation, early information about the planned measures is desirable. In this way, problems can be identified and solved in advance. Personal contact with the patient is indispensable. At the first appointment, which should already take place in the hospital when the patient is transferred from the inpatient area, both the medical and the social anamnesis (living situation, relatives) are taken. The patient or the relatives/ caregivers are also informed about the patient's right of choice (choice of a provider, data protection guidelines for care), the course of the planned therapy measures, any costs incurred such as statutory co-payments and other questions are answered.

The care manager contacts the outpatient prescriber and clarifies further supply and prescription management. All relevant information is communicated promptly to all cooperation partners.

Depending on the agreement, the Care Manager trains the nursing staff of the outpatient nursing service, the inpatient nursing facilities and/or the patients and their relatives in the handling of medical devices to be used (instruction in accordance with MPBetreibV, § 5 Para.1 No. 2 MPBetreibV) (MPBetreibV 2020), the materials and explains special hygienic measures.

During the course of care, regular home visits and progress checks are carried out by the care manager. These are documented in writing and communicated to the prescriber. A 24-h on-call service ensures constant availability in technical emergencies.

An indispensable counterpart to the care manager is the homecare company's office processing and associated logistics. Various professional groups work closely together here to ensure timely care that complies with the guidelines of the health insurance companies. The maintenance of customer data on a central platform, the processing of orders from the field service, including prescription management, as well as enquiries to the cost units for reimbursement of services are the central tasks of the office service. In addition, the office staff acts as a back-up for the care manager in order to facilitate the smooth provision of care. Besides, orders are passed on from here to the other cooperation partners, e.g., the pharmacy.

9.1.4   Pharmacy

The infusions administered via the port represent pharmacy-required and usually also prescription drugs. In principle, every pharmacy is able to obtain the required finished medicinal products from its wholesaler and to hand them over to the patient after presentation of the prescription. However, if drugs are required that are individually tailored to the patient, the pharmacy must have special clean rooms for the production of the corresponding prescriptions. The condition and equipment as well as the validation of the clean rooms are described in the Pharmacy Operations Ordinance (ApBetrO), in the guidelines of the Federal Chamber of Pharmacists as well as in the QM manual of the pharmacy. Compliance with the specifications is regularly checked by the responsible official pharmacist. For example, the absence of germs and particles in the clean room and in the manufactured products must be regularly confirmed by external companies. Special airlock systems and clean room benches with corresponding ventilation systems as well as trained pharmaceutical personnel are necessary to guarantee the absence of germs and particles in the product (ApBetrO 2020).

They are in constant contact with the care manager in order to design user-friendly therapy options for the patient. Pharmaceutical knowledge is also indispensable in the setting of pain and nutrition therapies as well as antibiotics. Stability requests and the development of therapy alternatives require close communication between physician and pharmacist.

9.1.5 Health Insurances

All partners of care in the outpatient sector are bound by the specifications and deadlines of the patient's health insurance company. In order to avoid recourse and retaxation during or after the end of therapy, the assumption of costs and prescribability should be sufficiently clarified before treatment or delivery. This often poses logistical and time problems for the parties providing care, as the actual need for therapy is only clarified shortly before the patient is discharged.

The decisive factor for the assumption of costs is § 12 SGB V paragraph (1): "The services must be sufficient, appropriate and economical; they must not exceed the extent of what is necessary. Services that are not necessary or uneconomical cannot be claimed by insured persons, may not be provided by the service providers and may not be approved by the health insurance funds."

The basis for the medical prescription of the therapy is the guideline of the Joint Federal Committee in the respective currently valid version (§ 92 para. 1 SGB V). This guideline is binding for all service providers/contractual partners (specialized trade, pharmacies, nursing services, medical profession) and assigns the decision on the prescription to the physicians (prescription authority). Despite the prescription sovereignty, the provision of medical aids and care by a nursing service often requires separate approval by the health insurance fund. The latter has according to § 13 Abs. 13a SGB V after request entrance up to 3 weeks time to approve the claim. A period of time that forces providers in practice to deliver care at their own expense or at the expense of the patient without prior approval in order to ensure uninterrupted care from the day of discharge.

> **Practical Tip**
> - Due to the high amount of co-payments, the exemption limit is often reached quickly!
> - Educate patient and get exemption limit clarified.
> - Any additional payment made can also be declared as an "extraordinary burden" in the tax return.
> - After signing a declaration of assignment, many private health insurance companies allow contractual partners to bill them directly. This is an enormous relief for patients and relatives, who are often greatly disturbed by the high bills.

9.1.6 Outpatient Care Service

Ambulatory care services play a central role in the qualified care of patients with port systems. As a rule, they are most frequently on site and are the first point of contact for patients and relatives.

Generally, the patient is taken over after notification by the hospital, the practicing physician/MVZ or the homecare company. In the admission interview, all relevant medical and social data are recorded anamnestically and the measures necessary for the care are initiated. The commissioning of the nursing service becomes effective with the issuing of the "prescription for home nursing care" by the prescribing doctor and the approval of the services by the responsible health insurance company; in addition to the relevant diagnoses, the prescription contains the services to be provided as well as the start, frequency and duration of the measures. All prescribable measures are listed in the "List of prescribable home nursing measures (List of services)—Annex to the Home Nursing Guideline in accordance with § 92 Paragraph 1 Sentence 2 No. 6 and Paragraph 7 SGB V". Measures not listed there, e.g. port puncture, may be performed by registered nurses with appropriate formal (theoretical) and material (practical) qualifications according to the "Transfer Guideline of the G-BA" of March 21, 2012, but are not reimbursable.

In this case, the port puncture is often delegated to the care manager or special palliative care teams. Since April 1, 2007, patients with corresponding eligibility requirements have been entitled to Specialized Outpatient Palliative Care (SAPV) in accordance with § 132d Para. 2 and § 37b of the German Social Code, Book V (SGB V). However, there is currently no uniform nationwide procedure and remuneration for SAPV.

9.1.7 Inpatient Care Facilities/Assisted Living Facilities

In recent years, the number of patients supplied via a port system who are residents of inpatient care facilities or assisted living centers has been steadily increasing. Section 84 (1) SGB XI regulates the assessment principles: "Nursing rates are the fees paid by nursing home residents or their payers for the partial or full inpatient nursing services provided by the nursing home as well as for care and, insofar as there is no entitlement to nursing care pursuant to Section 37 of the Fifth Book, for medical treatment care" (SGB IX 2017). This means that in inpatient care facilities, the fees for port care by registered nursing staff are often already included in the nursing rate, depending on the extent of the necessary treatment care measures. In assisted living facilities, on the other hand, Section 37 of the German Social Code, Book V—Home Nursing Care—applies.

In the case of palliative care, hospice and palliative care in nursing homes or homes for the elderly, the health insurance fund bears the costs for Specialized Outpatient Palliative Care (SAPV), which comprises "medical and nursing services, including their coordination, in particular for pain therapy and symptom control" (SGB V 2016).

The materials and medications required for a port treatment are prescribed by the attending general practitioner or specialist, and are usually supplied by a cooperating homecare company and/or a specialized pharmacy.

9.2   Types of Supply

9.2.1   Parenteral Nutrition

In contrast to peripheral vascular access, infusion with a high nutrient concentration is possible via central venous access. With peripheral vascular access, the administration of hyperosmolar nutrient solution mixtures with an osmolarity >800 mosm/l leads to vein irritation (Jauch et al. 2008).

A medical and social anamnesis, current laboratory values and the current nutritional status are to be requested. Specialized nutritionists calculate the alimentation regime taking into account all dietarily relevant parameters and the stability of the nutritional solution mixture. Particularly in the palliative care setting, a risk-benefit assessment is necessary because the amount of nutrients to be administered must be able to be metabolized. The guidelines of the respective professional societies must be observed here (Körner et al. 2008).

In practice, all-in-one (AIO) nutrient solution mixtures have gained acceptance over single-component supply due to the lower risk of infection (Löser 2017). AIO nutrient solution mixtures are available as industrially produced standard formulations, but also as formulations individually composed for the patient and produced in the clean room laboratory of a pharmacy (so-called "compounding").

The advantages of standard formulations are their longer shelf life and easy storage at room temperature, while compounding sachets have a limited shelf life (6–28 days from the date of manufacture, depending on the composition and starting solution) and must be stored in the refrigerator. On the other hand, compounding allows for a patient-specific composition of both macro- and micronutrients.

In principle, nutrient solutions are not carrier solutions for drugs. Adding drugs to the nutrient solution mixtures can lead to precipitation of the drug and to breaking of the emulsion present in nutrient solution mixtures.

The use of a feeding pump provides greater assurance of consistent substrate delivery compared to gravity feeding, optimizing tolerance.

> **Practical Tip**
> - Nutrition must usually be infused for at least 10 h → overnight application recommended.

(continued)

- Maintain patient mobility through use of feeding pumps and backpack system.
- Consider storage possibilities at the patient (quantities).
- Do not store nutrient solution mixtures (standard products) and materials on floors with underfloor heating.

9.2.2 Pain Therapy

Pump-controlled pain therapies via port systems have become an indispensable part of modern pain therapy. In contrast to oral medication or injections, they enable a continuous basic therapy with pain medication that can be adapted to the current conditions at any time by changing the drip rate. In addition, demand-oriented bolus administration enables the therapy of pain peaks and breakthrough pain. When switching from oral or transdermal pain therapy to intravenous administration, the current need for intravenous analgesic per 24 h is determined using conversion tables that take into account the different routes of application.

Depending on the patient's symptoms, monotherapies or mixed therapies with two or more components are used here. Opioid and non-opioid analgesics as well as co-analgesics from the groups of antidepressants, antipsychotics, parasympatholytics are used here. Each time another drug is added, as well as when adjusting the dose, the compatibility of the individual drugs with each other must be carefully checked. Any crystallization and precipitation can endanger the port system and severely reduce the effectiveness of pain therapy.

In outpatient pain therapy, small and handy pumps are used so that the patient retains the greatest possible mobility.

Practical Tip
- Observe shelf life! Stability is significantly higher with monotherapies than with mixed therapies.
- Check venting of medication bags and systems before connection.

9.2.3 Administration of Medication

Central venous port systems offer significant advantages over other venous accesses, especially for cytostatic therapy in the field of drug-based tumor therapy: They are easy and frequent to puncture, can be used for a long time (over years), allow long infusion durations and the administration of substances with high tissue toxicity. The therapies can almost always be performed on an outpatient basis (Schweigert 2016).

Systemic infections often require the administration of an anti-infective several times a day over a period of several weeks. With an available port system, the patient can be treated on an outpatient basis and recover in a home environment if the port needle is in place, all therapy partners cooperate well and, last but not least, the drug is well tolerated. Port systems are also being used more and more frequently as an "emergency access" in the field of acute medication, e.g., for neurological diseases.

> **Practical Tip**
> - After administration of medication, rinse port well with 20–50 ml 0.9% NaCl solution
> - For ports not in constant use, regular flushing as ordered by a doctor, usually every 4–6 weeks

9.3 Basic Rules for Outpatient Care

9.3.1 Patient

"Education takes away fears." This sentence sounds simple, but putting it into practice seems difficult at times. The prerequisite for this is the establishment of a stable relationship of trust with the patient and their relatives. This requires good communication between all those involved in the care process. Knowing the patient's level of knowledge and education about his or her disease, prognosis and therapy and, based on this, coordinated therapy options give the patient security and a positive attitude for the implementation of the planned measures. Patients should have as precise an overview as possible of the course of therapy in order to be able to ask specific questions and if necessary act in case deviations occur during care.

Many patients are anxious. They often have a long and complex treatment history behind them, especially in the palliative field. In addition, they have often experienced highly stressful side effects of the therapies. The question of the meaningfulness of further treatments and the fear of the unknown are therefore always present. The subjective security of the hospital with specialists available at all times is missing in the outpatient area. A pronounced sensitivity, understanding and conveying of security reassurance towards the patient and his relatives in communication and practical work are indispensable foundations of successful care.

The wish for more rest, expressed again and again by patients, is to be included and implemented in the therapy options and plans, if possible, through proper planning, organization and realization.

9.3.2   Outpatient Care Service/Homecare Company

The basis of patient care is a comprehensive medical and social anamnesis. The scope of care is determined and the planned operating times are discussed with the patients. It is clarified which service provider will take over the 24-h on-call service and how its availability is guaranteed. The registered nursing staff of both service providers support the patients and relatives during the entire care period.

▶   A prerequisite for qualified care is that only competent and regularly
     trained personnel who are familiar with both the materials and the care
     of port systems and who can demonstrate both formal (theoretical) and
     material (practically acquired) qualifications are employed.

It appears problematic that there is currently no uniform training and care standard. Different providers (manufacturers, homecare companies, clinics) train partly very different standards (gloves vs. non-touch technique, drawing up ampoules with vs. without cannula, etc.) to different extents. A standard developed in quality management and described in the quality manual should be made binding for all employees in every outpatient care service (Schweigert 2016). Regular quality audits, also in the practical work, ensure a high quality of care. The aim here is to uncover potential for improvement.

The different material requirements resulting from different standards must be clarified by regular communication between the outpatient nursing service and the care manager about required material, possible additional consumption and changes.

It should be noted that additional services, e.g., the application of taurolidine, are usually not included in the standard and must be trained separately. Legal questions arise due to the various and in some cases little-used resolutions and guidelines of the G-BA, which in some cases do not remunerate the services of home nursing (e.g. port puncture), but allow them in other places (transferability of medical activities to registered nurses) (see Chap. 4).

9.3.3   Hygiene

Adherence to simple hygiene measures in port care prevents contamination and significantly reduces the risk of infection (see Chap. 3). Always ensure that aseptic work is carried out first and then septic work. The material for both areas of activity must be stored separately.

It should already be clarified during the admission interview that liquid soap and clean (disposable) towels are available for washing hands. Jewelry should be taken off. Gloves should be worn for all activities at the port. Disinfectants should be used in accordance with the manufacturer's instructions and disinfection times should be strictly adhered to. The working environment should be as clean as possible; a sterile underlay ensures this, at least for all materials required. Windows and doors in the therapy room must be kept closed during the treatment. Pets are to be removed from the therapy room. All persons in the room should wear a mouth guard during preparation and port fitting. As described in Sect. 9.2, only AIO nutrient mixtures should be used for parenteral nutrition. As little manipulation as possible should be carried out on the port and the materials required; all non-sterile connections, e.g., connectors, should be disinfected before each procedure. For example, 20 ml syringes and ampoules can be used instead of the standard 10 ml syringes and ampoules for a larger flush volume, as this halves the number of manipulations. Any unnecessary port puncture should be avoided, as this increases the risk of infection and can endanger the port system due to incorrect punctures (Hofmann 2016). The puncture site should be cleared of clothing over a large area to avoid contamination.

The patient should lie as still as possible during the fitting at the port in order not to contaminate the connection points and materials by movements; if necessary, new materials should be used.

The port needle line should be fixed as far away as possible from other, septic accesses (tracheostoma, stoma) with a universal fixation/plaster; at the same time, this prevents mechanical traction on the port needle (Schulz-Stübner and Simon 2016).

During all activities at the port, it must be ensured that the system remains locked by closing the clamp or using a connector. Missing connection systems, e.g., after therapies in the doctor's office or clinic, must be replaced promptly by the registered nursing staff.

Basic Rules
- Avoid unnecessary port punctures and manipulations
- Wash hands
- Wear gloves
- Nitrile gloves can be disinfected according to DIN EN 374
- Use sterile gloves for port puncture
- Create a large work area and avoid contamination by removing the patient's outer clothing
- Observe disinfection times
- Plan workflows: first aseptic work, then septic work
- Separate storage of materials for aseptic and septic care

▶   **Practical Tip**
Use 20 ml syringes and ampoules for larger rinsing volumes.

9.3.4 Complications

Occlusion

If the port is occluded, a maximum of three flushing attempts with isotonic saline solution in a 10 ml syringe are made, depending on the physician's instructions. In the absence of success, a visit to the clinic is necessary, because only there may a drug-assisted flushing attempt with urokinase be undertaken (Hofmann 2016; Sucker 2016).

Syringes with a volume smaller than 10 ml are not suitable for flushing due to the high pressure exerted on the port.

Infection

Caution is advised in case of redness and swelling as well as discharge of secretion from the puncture site. Inquire whether mechanical traction or pressure may have been applied to the puncture site. If this is denied, a port infection is likely. In this case, further port puncture should be discouraged and the prescribing physician should be informed promptly.

The same applies if chills or fever suddenly occur after the infusion connection. In this case, parenteral nutrition must be stopped immediately and the port must be flushed carefully and with a low volume to avoid occlusions. The prescribing physician must be informed immediately; this also applies to ongoing pain therapy.

Mechanical Problems

The most frequent mechanical complications in port care occur in the form of dislocation of the port needle due to accidental placement or stepping on the infusion system in mobile patients. The patients or their relatives are informed before the start of care whether immediate consultation with the outpatient nursing service or homecare company is necessary or whether the next intervention can be waited for; this depends on the type of therapy.

Due to missing non-return valves, blood may flow back through the port system into the infusion line in the case of gravity-fed supply. In this case, prompt flushing is always required to avoid occlusions.

In this instance of gravity feeds, the infusion speed can be increased or reduced or overridden by the position of the patient. Here, too, instruction of the patient is necessary for the case of need.

References

Apothekenbetriebsordnung in der Fassung der Bekanntmachung vom 26. September 1995 (BGBl. I S. 1195), diezuletzt durch Artikel 10 des Gesetzes vom 3. Juni 2021 (BGBl. I S. 1309) geändert worden ist

Gemeinsamer Bundesausschuss (2012) Richtlinie des Gemeinsamen Bundesausschusses über die Festlegung ärztlicher Tätigkeiten auf Berufsangehörige der Alten- und Krankenpflege zur selbständigen Ausübung von Heilkunde im Rahmen von Modellvorhaben nach § 63 Abs. 3c SGB V (Richtlinie nach § 63 Abs. 3c SGB V) in der Fassung vom 20. Oktober 2011, veröffentlicht im Bundesanzeiger Nr. 46 (S. 1128) vom 21. März 2012 und Nr. 50 (S. 1228) vom 28. März 2012 in Kraft getreten am 22. März 2012. Bundesanzeiger, Köln

Gemeinsamer Bundesausschuss (2015a) Bekanntmachung eines Beschlusses des Gemeinsamen Bundesausschusses über eine Änderung der Arzneimittel-Richtlinie (AM-RL): Entlassmanagement vom 17.Dezember 2015, veröffentlicht im Bundesanzeiger BAnZ AT 15.03.2016 B5 am 15.März 2016 in Kraft getreten am 16. März 2016. Bundesanzeiger, Köln

Gemeinsamer Bundesausschuss (2015b) Richtlinie des Gemeinsamen Bundesausschusses über die Verordnung von häuslicher Krankenpflege (Häusliche Krankenpflege-Richtlinie) in der Neufassung vom 17. September 2009, veröffentlicht im Bundesanzeiger 9. Februar 2010, in Kraft getreten am 10. Februar 2010, zuletzt geändert am 17. Dezember 2015, veröffentlicht im Bundesanzeiger AT 18.03.2016B3 vom 18. März 2016 in Kraft getreten am 19. März 2016. Bundesanzeiger, Köln

Hofmann HAF (2016) Postoperative Betreuung nach Portimplantationen. In: Hennes R, Hofmann HAF (Hrsg) Ports. Versorgungsstandards, Implantationstechniken, Portpflege. Springer, Berlin, S 97–108

Jauch KW et al (2008) 7: Technik und Probleme der Zugänge in der parenteralen Ernährung. In: Deutche Gesellschaft für Ernährungsmedizin e. V. (Hrsg) DGEM-Leitlinien Enterale und Parenterale Ernährung. Kurzfassung. Thieme, Stuttgart, S 118–123

Körner U et al (2008) Anhang 2: Ökonomische, rechtliche und ethische Aspekte. In: Deutsche Gesellschaft für Ernährungsmedizin e.V. (Hrsg) DGEM-Leitlinien Enterale und Parenterale Ernährung. Kurzfassung. Thieme, Stuttgart, S 118–123

Leitlinie der Bundesapothekenkammer zur Qualitätssicherung: Aseptische Herstellung und Prüfung applikationsfertiger Parenteralika. Stand der Revision: 13.11.2019

Löser C (2017) Parenterale Ernährung—Grundlagen und Durchführung. Aktuelle Ernährungsmedizin 1:53–74

Schulz-Stübner S, Simon A (2016) Infektionen in der Portchirurgie, Prophylaxe, Therapie, Hygienestandards. In: Hennes R, Hofmann HAF (Hrsg) Ports. Versorgungsstandards, Implantationstechniken, Portpflege. Springer, Berlin, S 151–160

Schweigert M (2016) Portanwendung in der Chemotherapie und für sonstige Medikationen. In: Hennes R, Hofmann HAF (Hrsg) Ports. Versorgungsstandards, Implantationstechniken, Portpflege. Springer, Berlin, S 111–117

Sozialgesetzbuch (SGB) (2019) Sozialgesetzbuch (SGB XI) Elftes Buch Soziale Pflegeversicherung. Zuletzt geändert durch Art. 2 G vom 21.12.2019

Sozialgesetzbuch (SGB) (2020) Sozialgesetzbuch (SGB V) Fünftes Buch Gesetzliche Krankenversicherung. Zuletzt geändert durch Art. 5 G vom 10.2.2020

Sucker C (2016) Gerinnung, Thrombosen, Okklusionen in der Portchirurgie. In: Hennes R, Hofmann HAF (Hrsg) Ports. Versorgungsstandards, Implantationstechniken, Portpflege. Springer, Berlin, S 161–173

Verordnung über das Errichten, Betreiben und Anwenden von Medizinprodukten (Medizinprodukte-Betreiberverordnung—MPBetreibV) (2020) § 5 Besondere Anforderungen. https://www.gesetze-im-internet.de/mpbetreibv/. Zugegriffen: 11.3.2020

Care of Special Patient Groups

10

Julia Winkler, Debora Stern, Bianka Walter, and Damaris Weeber

Summary Handling a port system is a particular challenge for the caregiver, especially for cachectic or obese patients. The resulting difference in tissue thickness between the port chamber and the skin surface requires an adjustment of the port care.

Particularly in oncological patients who are dependent on a port during further treatment, weight fluctuations occur frequently due to malnutrition or cortisone medication, for example.

Consequently, port care must be provided by the caring healthcare professional in a manner that takes into account and continually adjusts for cachexia, obesity, and weight fluctuations.

10.1 Cachectic Patients

Due to malnutrition caused by illness or treatment-related nutritional disorders, cachexia may be present when a port is inserted and severe weight loss may occur during the course of treatment of an illness. This leads to the fact that there is only a thin layer of tissue above the port chamber, i.e. between the port chamber and the skin surface, and thus there is no "cushion" or support for the port needle.

Choosing the right needle length—in this case the smallest possible—offers the chance to insert the largest part of the needle into the port chamber and thus achieve a stable fit.

J. Winkler (✉) · B. Walter
Department of Hematology, Oncology and Rheumatology, Heidelberg University Hospital, Heidelberg, Germany
e-mail: Julia.Winkler@med.uni-heidelberg.de; Bianka.Walther@med.uni-heidelberg.de

D. Stern · D. Weeber
Department of Pediatric Oncology, Hematology, Immunology and Pneumology, Heidelberg University Hospital, Heidelberg, Germany
e-mail: Deborah.Stern@med.uni-heidelberg.de; Damaris.Weeber@med.uni-heidelberg.de

© Springer-Verlag GmbH Germany, part of Springer Nature 2022
R. Hennes, G. Müller (eds.), *Port Care*,
https://doi.org/10.1007/978-3-662-64494-2_10

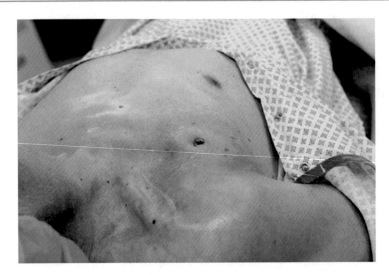

Fig. 10.1 Cachectic patient with extensive skin defect over the port chamber. (Source: Rodrian, University Hospital Heidelberg)

A port needle that is too large and therefore unstable can cause the puncture site to expand due to the constant movement. After the needle has been withdrawn, this prolongs wound healing and makes puncture more difficult, especially during direct re-puncturing.

Port needles differ in both length and lumen of the needle. Not all lengths are available with every diameter. The required lumen size of the port needle depends on the fluids to be administered through the port. For parenteral nutrition, the lumen should be at least 20 G.

Puncturing a port in a cachectic patient is a relatively simple task. The port chamber, although mostly flat (8–9 mm) models with small silicone membrane are chosen, is easily visible and palpable. However, this may favor the development of a stitch canal. Due to the optimal localization of the port chamber and the small diameter of the silicone membrane, many caregivers choose exactly the same puncture site, which then forms a puncture channel over time that no longer closes (Fig. 10.1).

▶   **Practical tip** As a preventive measure, it is advisable to consciously ensure that the port chamber is not only centrally punctured.

In addition to stabilizing the port needle, the tissue over the port chamber also has the function of "cushioning" the surface of the skin to relieve the pressure on the skin between the wing or retaining plate of the port needle and the port chamber. If the subcutis is too thin, a pressure sore with formation of necrosis by the port needle itself may occur. When applying the dressing, additional cushioning can be created by lining the port needle with sterile slit dressings. In addition, the fixation of the port needle with plaster should not be too tight in order not to increase the pressure of the port needle on the skin by the pull of the plaster.

In order to detect a possible strain ulcer as quickly as possible, the dressing must be changed every 48 h at the latest so that there is a clear view of the port needle and the skin.

It is useful to make the patient aware of all aspects of their port catheter. The nurse can actively inform them of the risks and ask about any pain or burning at the port site and also about the port environment.

If there is a strong weight loss in the period after the port implantation, the initially fitting reservoir becomes too large. The loss of tissue padding can lead to pressure sores in the skin, which can result in necrosis. In this case the port must be revised.

Prophylactically, an analysis of the nutritional status and a dietary consultation with evaluation should be performed in the early stage of treatment, however, not only because of a possible necrosis above the port, but mainly because of the generally high risk of tumor cachexia and the associated risks.

▶ Choosing the right port needle length ensures the greatest possible safety! Certain manufacturers offer port needles from 10 mm length.

10.2   Obese Patients

Too much tissue also influences the port placement and the later handling of the port catheter system. Similar risks exist not only for obese patients but also for women with large breasts. The causes of possible problems are the depth of the tissue and the greater movements or forces acting on the port catheter system, the port needle and the port environment.

Furthermore, the choice of a larger port body (12–13 mm) can compensate somewhat for the tissue depth. Placement is further sternal, where the subcutaneous fat pad is lowest (Fig. 5.5).

▶ **Practical tip** The obese patient, but also women with large breasts, should sit upright when puncturing the port in order to minimize the soft tissue over the port chamber. Evasive movements of the patient backwards during the needle insertion can be avoided by a seat with a firm and high back support.

▶ In order to present the port chamber even more clearly, the person is asked to take the shoulders back and stick out the chest. If possible, the same-sided arm can also be placed on the back and a deep breath taken just before the puncture.

The person performing the insertion can feel the port chamber better thanks to the above-mentioned measures and is therefore in a good position for the upcoming puncture. After the further preparations, the port should be fixed with three fingers during the maneuver to prevent it from slipping away.

The subsequent additional fixation of the port needle gives it a secure hold and thus prevents dislocation and associated extravasation during movement.

> ▶   **Practical tip** Any adhesive dressing over the sterile plaster should not be
>   pulled too tightly, as this can cause tension blisters.

If infusions are administered to the patient via infusomats, a recurring pressure alarm may indicate that the port needle is no longer correctly positioned in the cavity of the port chamber or that there is an occlusion in the port catheter. In this case, the position of the port needle must be checked and corrected if necessary.

> ▶   Due to the overall increased risk of extravasation in the obese patient
>   and the fact that extravasation is only detected at a late stage, the correct
>   position of the port needle is particularly important. The depth of the soft
>   tissue provides space for large amounts of fluid before extravasation
>   becomes visible externally.

One of the most important points in avoiding extravasation is the correct needle length. The responsible surgeon or nurse enters this into the port passport immediately after implantation of the port.

Before the start of each infusion, the correct position of the port needle is checked by aspiration of blood. For continuous infusions, intermediate checks should take place if the infusion content permits. A visual inspection of the thorax is also helpful to learn about the patient's anatomical features. This is repeated during the course of the infusions, paying particular attention to the comparison between the port side and the opposite side (Fig. 5.4).

For shorter and highly tissue toxic therapies, it is advisable to ask the patient to move as little as possible during this time. With the information about the risk, the patient receives the justification for this restriction and can help to detect extravasation early through self-observation.

The same applies directly after port implantation for early detection of bleeding or a hematoma, which can only be seen late due to the depth of the tissue. In addition to the vital parameters, the port area and, for comparison, the opposite side of the thorax should be inspected regularly during the first 2 days. Prophylactically, the surgical area can be cooled with cool packs after implantation. Sandbags, which are intended to exert mechanical compression of the wound area, are not tolerable for some patients after local anesthesia has worn off, especially if a port needle has been left intraoperatively for early use.

Obese people often have increased perspiration. Especially in oncology, however—can be erased, night sweats, fever and certain medications also cause augmented moisture of the skin. This loosens the bandage and thus the fixation of the port needle. In addition, the sweat and the exposure of the puncture site cause contamination underneath the port needle.

Therefore, a regular control of the dressing should be carried out, which can be done by the responsible caregiver as well as by the patient himself.

▶   **Practical tip** Sterile skin protection wipes (SKIN-PREP®), which improve the self-sealing properties of adhesive dressings, are available on the market.

In general, when puncturing the port, care should be taken to determine the direction in which the extension tube is discharged. This can be influenced directly after insertion by turning the port needle and keeping the end of the tube from slipping into the armpit and thus preventing the spread of germs.

▶   **Practical tip** The branch of the tube at the port needle should point in the direction of 8 o'clock and the tube section can also be tightened with a strip of plaster.

10.3   Patients with Systemic Diseases

Systemic diseases are diseases that affect an organ system. These can affect the skin, the muscles, the connective tissue, the bones, the central nervous system and the immune system, but also the hematopoietic and lymphatic system. Frequently, the use of a port system is indicated for these diseases due to therapy and supportive measures. However, the use of ports in patients with systemic diseases also poses special challenges. Those will be illustrated in the following using selected diseases as examples.

10.3.1 Hematological/Lymphatic Diseases

Malignant diseases of the hematopoietic and lymphatic systems represent a large group of systemic diseases. Using the example of leukemia, the special duty of care in handling the port is now to be demonstrated. Due to the defective maturation of the leukocytes, patients with leukemia suffer from a particular **risk of infection.** In addition, cytostatic therapy leads to further immunosuppression. When dealing with patients suffering from leukemia, and also with patients suffering from other systemic diseases, it is very important to reduce environmental germs to a minimum, as these pose a particular threat to the decreased immune defenses. This is done in everyday hospital life primarily through aseptic work on patients and strict adherence to hygiene guidelines.

Since these patients have very poor venous conditions due to both their underlying disease and the therapy (e.g. cortisone, cytostatics), the port represents a safe access for the therapy. All necessary therapeutic agents such as cytostatics, analgesics, antibiotics, parenteral nutrition solutions can be infused through the port. Careful handling of the port in patients with systemic diseases is particularly important.

The Following Principles Should Be Considered

- The indication for puncturing the port from a hygienic point of view must be strict, as a lying port needle always poses a risk of infection (e.g. for a single blood sample, puncture of a peripheral vein should be preferred)
- Port puncture is performed under sterile conditions (Sect. 5.4, 5.6)
- When puncturing, ensure that the tube is positioned in the 8 o'clock direction to avoid alignment in the axilla (spread of germs)
- Before each contact with the port system, hygienic hand disinfection is performed
- Disposable gloves are worn for self-protection
- When connecting or disconnecting infusion solutions, a sterile compress is placed underneath and the cone of the three-way stopcock is spray disinfected with an alcohol solution (e.g. Cutasept F®)
- When changing dressings, instruct patient not to talk and to turn head to the side (away from port)
- **Pay attention to the** maximum lying time of the needle (maximum 7 days)
- Daily check of the port environment (e.g. redness, swelling)
- Contaminations such as blood residues on the cone are to be removed with a sterile compress
- Guide the patient to self-observation (e.g. pain, swelling)
- Inform patient about proper handling of their port and encourage them to have only trained personnel handle their port

Practical Tip
- If fever or chills occur shortly after the port has been inserted, a port infection should always be considered! (see Chap. 5)
- For immunosuppressed patients, the rule is: as much manipulation as necessary, as little as possible!
- If the port is not used for more than 24 h, a port block with an antiseptic, e.g., taurolidine, should be performed in immunosuppressed patients.

In connection with leukemias, in addition to the risk of infection, the increased bleeding tendency should also be mentioned. **Thrombocytopenia** can occur as a side effect of the underlying disease and also as a consequence of cytostatic therapy.

Immediately after port implantation, the skin area may be bruised and swollen for a few days (Fig. 10.2). If necessary, this can be cooled with a cool pack.

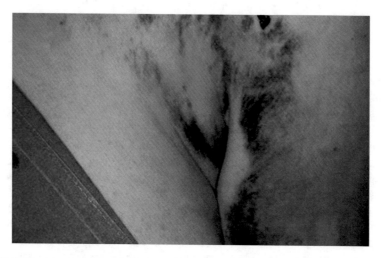

Fig. 10.2 Hematoma after port implantation. (Source: Rodrian, University Hospital Heidelberg)

▶   **Practical tip** In order to be able to use the port for the necessary therapy directly after implantation, it makes sense to leave the port needle in the operating theatre after the first piercing. This requires information to the surgeon. A puncture through the swollen, hematous tissue can be very painful or impossible.

Thrombocytopenia occasionally results in secondary bleeding at the needle puncture. The blood should always be removed during the twice-a-day dressing changes.

During bandage replacement care should be taken to keep the adhesive area as small as possible and to avoid skin folds under the dressing to prevent hematoma and petechiae.

▶   **Practice Tip** Due to thrombocytopenia, petechiae may occur under fixation and restraint.

10.3.2 Scleroderma

Scleroderma is a chronic inflammatory rheumatic disease. A special feature is the sclerosis of the connective tissue. Affected are the internal organs and vessels as well as the skin and subcutaneous tissue. This becomes hard and looses its elasticity.

Scleroderma is divided into a limited cutaneous and a diffuse form. In the limited form, there is thickening and hardening of the skin on the hands and feet, while in a diffuse manifestation the skin of the entire trunk and internal organs can be affected. A port is often necessary in the course of the disease, as the skin sclerosis makes it increasingly difficult to obtain safe central venous access.

Due to the nature of the skin, it is sometimes necessary to select an unusual site with as little affected skin as possible when implanting the port. Wound healing problems should be considered initially and controlled accordingly.

▶ **Practical tip** After initial implantation, the wound area must be checked regularly with particular attention to wound healing and suture dehiscence!

While in scleroderma the dermis (subcutis, dermis) hardens, the epidermis (epidermis) becomes thinner and more vulnerable. Rhagades and small fissures occur repeatedly due to the lack of elasticity and form entry points for infectious agents.

Another challenge is the adhesion of the adhesive surfaces. The plaster sticks poorly to sclerosed skin and at the same time the skin should not be additionally irritated by large adhesive surfaces. The port needle change must be individually designed depending on the skin status in the port area. It may be necessary to change the needle more frequently if the skin is irritated or the dressing is dislocated due to limited fixation possibilities. When removing the port plaster, special care must be taken not to damage the epidermis.

▶ **Practical tip** Port plasters must be removed with particular care and attention to avoid skin lesions.

If the skin over or around the port in a patient with scleroderma is very hardened, care must be taken to apply appropriate pressure when puncturing the port. The use of a longer needle may also be useful if the skin is very thickened.

▶ **Practical tip** A courageous puncturing of the port through thick and hardened skin can support the success of the puncture.

Port Care for Children

11

Heiko Riemke

Summary Already in infancy and toddlerhood a port is a safe venous access system. Due to the agility of children, the fixation of the needle is very important. The tube system must also be checked regularly and, if necessary, replaced more frequently. Complications must be recognized in time and eliminated as quickly as possible. Expressions of pain by young patients should always be taken seriously and the causes should be investigated.

11.1 Indications for Port Placement in Children

- Chemotherapy
- Parenteral nutrition
- As "emergency access", when quick action is necessary (e.g. derailment of metabolic patients)
- Poor vein conditions, if regular infusions or blood sampling must be performed
- Long-term administration of intravenous drugs
- Long-term high-percentage glucose administration in metabolic patients
- Substitution of immunoglobulins in immunological diseases
- Pain therapy in the palliative situation

H. Riemke (✉)
Center for Pediatric and Adolescent Medicine, Department of Gynecology, Department of Dermatology, Heidelberg University Hospital, Heidelberg, Germany
e-mail: Heiko.Riemke@med.uni-heidelberg.de

© Springer-Verlag GmbH Germany, part of Springer Nature 2022
R. Hennes, G. Müller (eds.), *Port Care*,
https://doi.org/10.1007/978-3-662-64494-2_11

11.2   Size of the Port Chamber

With port implantation, the size and weight of the child determine the size of the port. It does not automatically have to be replaced with a larger one after a certain period of time. Rather, the growth and weight gain of the child determine this. The following port sizes can be distinguished:

Baby port	Approx. 2.5 g
Child port	4–6 g
Adolescents/Adults	8–10 g

Different port chamber sizes are shown in Fig. 5.5.

11.3   Port Location in Children

There are different options for port placement in both children and adults. The most common port placement in children is below the subclavian.

11.3.1 Localizations

- Subcutaneously under the right or left clavicle
- Venae section of the cephalic or subclavian vein; if this is not possible, the external or internal jugular vein can also be used
- V. saphena magna: Placement in the groin
- V. basilica: inner side of the upper arm (flat port chamber)
- Tip of the catheter should be in the superior vena cava, in front of the right atrium

11.3.2 Port Passport

After the port has been implanted, each patient receives a port ID card. The ID card must be carried by each patient or the parents so that immediate action can be taken without delay in the event of an emergency.

The following items are included in the emergency ID card:

- Instructions for possible emergency measures
- Personal data of the port holder
- Implanting doctor
- Port designation (manufacturer, model, size)
- Batch number
- Site of the port chamber
- Catheter position

11.4 Postoperative Monitoring

11.4.1 Monitoring on the Ward

Postoperative monitoring usually takes place during an inpatient stay. Monitoring (monitoring of blood pressure, pulse, temperature, oxygen saturation) and pain therapy are the most important aspects. Regular dressing checks and assessment of the surgical site are also part of this. If the port is punctured, infusions must be administered continuously, otherwise thrombosis may occur in the port cannula/tube. Even at this stage, care must be taken to ensure that the port tube is well restrained, as children are often very agile and it is also not certain whether a child will accept the port immediately. To avoid disconnection of the tube system, all screw caps on the infusion are checked again and again. In addition, all screw connections of the tube system close to the patient are wrapped with a sterile swab.

11.4.2 Change of Dressing

The dressing of the port must be renewed regularly, at least every 2 days. In case of soiling, soaking or loosening of the dressing, a bandage replacement must be carried out correspondingly earlier. For newly implanted ports, the first change of dressing is performed together with a physician. At each dressing change replacement, check for needle dislocation and signs of infection.

▶ **Practical tip** Good fixation of the port tube or infusion line prevents disconnection of the system and pulling out or slipping of the port chamber.

11.5 Puncturing the Port

11.5.1 In Principle

Do not puncture the port if shortness of breath, chest pain, palpitations, signs of infection (redness, warmth, tenderness, swelling, pain) and skin reactions occur. In this case, you should consult the nearest physician.

Each port in place must be sterilely maintained and punctured under aseptic conditions to avoid possible complications such as infection. A needle change is required after 5–7 days at the latest. For the puncture of a port catheter only special port needles with spoon cut (curved or straight shape) may be used.

▶   The chamber size determines the size of the port needle. The needle size
     is noted in the port ID card. For children, a needle size of 19–24 G is
     usually used.

Do not use syringes smaller than 10 ml to flush the tubing system or port needle
(risk of overpressure in the port system, which can cause the tube to rupture or the
membrane to blow off).

The initial puncture is performed by an experienced physician, further punctures
can be performed by trained personnel or parents. There must be a daily inspection of
the port environment, the position of the port needle and the dressing.

11.5.2 Materials Needed

- Sterile pad
- Hand disinfectant
- Skin disinfectant
- Sterile and non-sterile gloves
- Mouthguard
- Sterile compresses
- 2 syringes à 10 ml NaCl 0.9%
- Port cannula (appropriate size)
- Three-way stopcock with extension and sealing plug
- Disposal box

11.5.3 Dressing

- Single use slit compress 7.5 × 7.5 cm or for babies 5.5 × 5.5 cm
  - Single use compress 7.5 × 7.5 cm or for babies 5.5 × 5.5 cm
  - Fixomull
  - Leucoplast

11.5.4 Preparation of the Patient

Care should be taken that windows and doors are closed. The child should be
informed about the planned procedure depending on its age and should lie comfortably. His face should always be positioned on the side facing away from the port.
With smaller children, the port should be punctured with at least two people, if
possible. One person fixes the child and thus enables the other person to puncture the
port sterilely and professionally.

If the port is used continuously, the puncture sites must be varied each time the
needle is changed, otherwise punching defects of the skin may occur.

11.5.5 Puncture of the Port Chamber

- Hand disinfection
- Put on non-sterile gloves and mouth guard
- Set up sterile tray including the required material
- Disinfection of the puncture area
- Skin disinfection according to the principle "spray—wipe—spray—wipe—spray—let it take effect"
- Remove gloves and disinfect hands again
- Put on sterile gloves
- Venting of the port needle with 10 ml NaCl 0.9%
- Palpate the port chamber and fix the port with thumb and index finger → while doing so, gently stretch the skin over the port chamber
- Have the patient look in the opposite direction or fix the children in this position
- Remove needle guard and hold port needle securely in place
- Puncture perpendicularly to the membrane of the port up to the needle stop
- Open the clamp of the port needle
- Aspiration test, if not possible, rinse with 10 ml NaCl 0.9%
- Another aspiration attempt
- Rinse again with 10 ml NaCl 0.9%
- Either: Screw on the sealing plug
- Or: Connect infusion therapy

11.5.6 Fixation of the Port

With children, the fixation or restraint of the port is very important in order to prevent the port needle from slipping/pulling out. Since the infusion tubing and thus also the port needle can quickly be pulled during playing and romping while the infusion is running, it must be fixed securely and in a manner suitable for children. It helps to cover the port needle with a small sterile compress and fix it with an adhesive bandage.

▶ **Practical tip** The restraining/fixing with children is carried out with plasters. Take about 10 cm depending on the size of the child, place the tube on the adhesive surface and then cross the strips over the tube and stick the ends to the outside.

11.5.7 Removal of the Port Needle

- In case of longer lay time, change of needle every 5–7 days
- Flush the port with 10 ml NaCl 0.9%
- Secure port with two fingers and out port needle with other hand

- Safely dispose of the port needle in the designated disposal box
- Skin disinfection of the puncture site with Octenisept and dressing with sterile wound plaster

11.5.8 Blocking the Port

The port is blocked with approx. 4–5 ml NaCl 0.9%, regardless of the dead space volume of the port. In immunocompromised patients or for port rehabilitation, blocking with Taurolock is recommended (as ordered by the physician).

11.6   Supply and Control

11.6.1 General

Depending on the age of the patient, it is important to educate the child well about dressing changes and needle replacement. The smaller the child, the more care and attention is needed when fixing the needle and tubing system.

Even the puncture in the skin means pain and therefore stress for many children. For this reason, a local anaesthetic for the skin should be used for each needle change. Emla ointment or Emla plasters are suitable for this purpose (for individual doses, see Table 11.1). In newborns and infants up to 2 months of age, the application time is a maximum of 1 h, from 3 to 11 months a maximum of 4 h. After the

Table 11.1 Dosage of Emla "R" Ointment for local anaesthesia

Age	Single dose	Reaction time/special features
Babies 0–2 months	Up to 1 g cream on max. 10 cm^2 skin	Do not apply for more than 1 h, only once in 24 h
Babies 3–11 months	Up to 2 g cream on max. 20 cm^2 skin	Application time approx. 1 h, max. 4 h. Maximum 2 doses at intervals of 12 h within 24 h
Toddlers 1–5 years	Up to 10 g cream on max. 100 cm^2 skin	Application time approx. 1 h, max. 5 h
Children 6–11 years	Up to 20 g cream on max. 200 cm^2 skin	Application time approx. 1 h, max. 5 h
Adolescents from 12 years and adults	– About 1.5 g cream per 10 cm^2 skin area – About 2 g cream for blood sampling (venipuncture) – Approximately 1.5–2 g per 10 cm^2 of skin for use in skin grafts during a hospital stay – Approximately 1 g of cream per 10 cm^2 of skin for use on freshly shaved skin, e.g., for laser hair removal (self-application by the patient)	60 g of cream per 600 cm^2 of skin area (this corresponds to an area of 30 × 20 cm, i.e., approximately the size of a DIN A4 sheet)

application of Emla in newborns and infants up to 3 months of age, the preparation may only be used again after 12 h.

11.6.2 With Needle Lying

The drip rate of the infusion with the needle in place is at least 2 ml and a maximum of 500 ml per hour. Showering can be performed without problems with a foil dressing (e.g., Tegaderm or Opsite foil).

The port environment should be inspected daily for signs of infection and pain. In addition, the position of the needle and the dressing must be checked every day. Secure fixation of the port needle is especially important in children. To prevent the port needle from being pulled out, the infusion tube or port tubing should be restrained. In daily handling, disconnections should be kept to an absolute minimum to avoid any infections or germ introduction.

11.6.3 With the Port Shut Down

If the port needle is not in place, showering can take place once wound healing is complete. If wound healing is not yet complete, a foil dressing should also be applied and then the dressing should be changed.

11.7   Complications

11.7.1 General Complications

- Infection
- Hematoma
- Fluid accumulation (extravasation) under the skin
- Hematoma in the port pocket (small → no intervention, large → surgery)
- Infection of the port pocket (swelling, redness)
- Thrombotic occlusion
- System infection
- Skin necrosis
- Catheter leakage
- Dislocation of the catheter

11.7.2 Wound Monitoring

Wound healing problems at the port can occur time and again. Therefore, proper skin and wound monitoring is very important. The skin around the port, but also the surgical wound and the pathway of the port catheter are observed. The first signs of a wound healing disorder may be redness, swelling, overheating or pain.

Other signs of a wound healing disorder or infection may include:

- Reddened or swollen skin around the wound
- Wound area warmer than other areas
- Secretion leaks from the wound
- Gaping wound edges
- Increasing pain
- Fever

Further Reading

Haeder L (2013) Indikation, Technik und Komplikationen der Portimplantation. In: Der Chirurg. Springer, Berlin
Zernikow B (2013) Palliativversorgung von Kindern, Jugendlichen und jungen Erwachsenen, 2 Aufl. Springer, Dordrecht

Documentation, Patient Counseling and Information

Margit Benz

Summary Das Deutsche Patienteninformationsgesetz (The German Patient Information Act) of February 2013 obliges the treating physician to explain to the patient "in an understandable manner at the beginning of the treatment and, if necessary, in the course of the treatment, all circumstances essential for the treatment, in particular the diagnosis, the probable health development, the therapy and the measures to be taken during and after the therapy".

Informing the patient, both about the course of treatment and about the actual surgical procedure, is of fundamental importance from both a medical and a legal point of view. A clear and transparent presentation of the medical content and procedures must be communicated to the patient in a comprehensible manner. This is all the more important as little objective and medically factually correct information can be found through the digital media. For patients who have received a port and their accompanying relatives, questions arise again and again in the daily handling of the port. In order to provide a service in this area, the Heidelberg Port Center has collected patients' questions and created a port information brochure that provides the relevant education on the organizational process—from instruction to implantation of the port—as well as explaining how to handle the port in the further course of treatment.

Based on the experience of the Heidelberg Port Centre at the Surgical University Hospital, the third new version of the port brochure has now been published as information for patients and their relatives. The very positive feedback shows that there is a high demand for clarification among patients and their relatives. The brochure explains in a clear way what a port catheter is and which areas of application there are. Pictures and graphics illustrate the data.

In addition to the basic explanation on the structure and function of a port catheter (Fig. 12.1), the organizational procedure of port surgery is also outlined (Fig. 12.2).

M. Benz (✉)
Surgical Clinic and Clinic for Anaesthesiology, Heidelberg University Hospital, Heidelberg, Germany
e-mail: Margit.Benz@med.uni-heidelberg.de

© Springer-Verlag GmbH Germany, part of Springer Nature 2022
R. Hennes, G. Müller (eds.), *Port Care*,
https://doi.org/10.1007/978-3-662-64494-2_12

INTRODUCTION

What is a port catheter?

The port catheter (short: port) is a permanent access to the venous or arterial blood circulation located in the subcutaneous fatty tissue. The port consists of a chamber with a thick silicone membrane and an attached tube made of polyurethane or silicone.

The small chamber can either be made of plastic, plastic-coated titanium, solid titanium or a combination with ceramic. The port catheter is implanted during a surgical procedure.

Access to the bloodstream is established by piercing the silicone membrane. Either blood can be withdrawn or a drug can be administered centrally in the body by infusion via the needle located in the port chamber

Fields of application

A port catheter is primarily used in tumor therapy. A port catheter is used primarily in tumor therapy, nutritional medicine, and pain management when frequent and safe venous or arterial access is required.

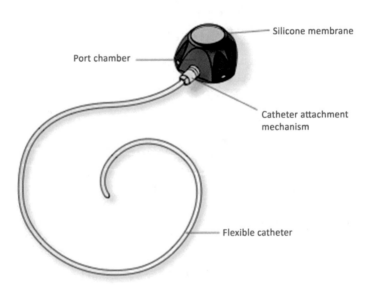

Fig. 12.1 Structure and function of a port catheter system. (Heidelberg University Hospital, "Wissenswertes rund um Ihren Port" September 2014)

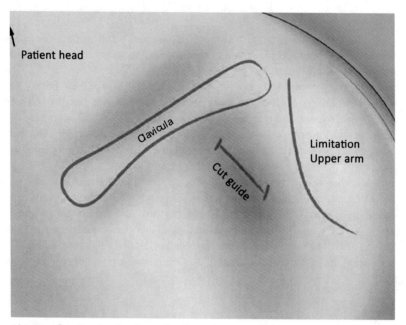

Planning for standardized port implantation

Outpatient surgery

In outpatient surgery, our nursing team will meet you and escort you to the operating room. It may be necessary to shave the surgical area. This may only be done immediately prior to surgery due to the risk of infection.

The surgeon will now administer the local anesthetic. This dose is usually sufficient to keep you pain-free throughout the operation. However, if you still feel pain, we can administer additional anesthetic at any time.

The position of your port catheter will be checked by x-ray during surgery.

There is an X-ray mat in the base of the operating table, so it will not be necessary to cover you with an additional lead apron.

Resting after the operation

After the operation you can leave the clinic immediately. However, if you still feel weak, you are welcome to rest a little longer in the day clinic

Fig. 12.2 Excerpt from the information brochure for patients and relatives on the surgical procedure. (Heidelberg University Hospital, "Wissenswertes rund um Ihren Port" September 2014)

The specific conditions of the Heidelberg Port Centre are described here; accordingly, each operating clinic can also pass on its specific information to the patient in order to ensure an optimized organizational procedure for the patient.

The format of the port brochure of the Heidelberg Port Centre can be requested from the Media Centre of Heidelberg University Hospital as a free download (Fig. 7.1).

Another major topic within the port brochure is wounds and wound monitoring. Here the patient is given specific recommendations on how to proceed in the event of problems or discomfort after the operation (Fig. 12.3).

The next set of topics relates to daily life, here the focus is on how life with the port works best. Questions about sporting activities, behavior in airports and when flying, personal hygiene and other areas are clarified.

It is important for port patients and their relatives to have a contact address and adequate contact persons to whom they can confidently turn with their questions. A daily port consultation is held at the Heidelberg Port Centre.

Along with the written and verbal information about the surgical procedure and the course of treatment, which is supported by the port brochure, the development of a so-called port letter is very helpful. This letter provides information about the surgical procedure with specific details about the catheters used, the implantation site and the type of skin closure. Furthermore, the contact details are given in it, Fig. 12.4 shows the port letter of Universitätsklinikum Heidelberg (Heidelberg University Hospital).

[12] UNIVERSITÄTSKLINIKUM **HEIDELBERG**

YOUR WOUND

After port implantation, your skin is usually closed with an absorbable suture or by skin glue. This has the advantage that you do not have to go to the doctor to have your stitches removed.

If your chemotherapy begins in the next few days, we will close your skin with sutures and insert a gripper. This will reduce the risk of wound healing problems.

Wound monitoring and care

Your surgical wound will also be covered with a plaster. You can leave this in place for two days. If you wish to shower during this time, we ask you to cover the wound with a waterproof plaster. You can get this plaster in any pharmacy. After the 3rd day you may shower without a bandage.

Has your wound changed?

The following observation criteria may be serious signs of a disturbance in the wound healing process:

- The surrounding skin is reddened.
- The surrounding skin is swollen.
- The immediate area is warmer than other areas.
- The wound secretes secretion
- The wound edges gape apart.
- The pain increases.
- You have a fever.

If one or more of these signs occur, you should contact our outpatient clinic.

If you notice anything unusual about the wound or if you are worried, you are welcome to call us or come by. (Tel: 06221 56-6220)

Fig. 12.3 Port brochure: Information on wound monitoring. (Heidelberg University Hospital, "Wissenswertes rund um Ihren Port" September 2014)

Here is the recommended procedure for the use of the port catheter by the trained physician or nursing staff according to the guidelines of Heidelberg University Hospital:

5.2.3 Puncture of the port catheter *(excerpt from the guidelines)*
- Hand disinfection.
- Put on non-sterile gloves and mouth protection. If none available, do not speak.
- Set up sterile tray including the required material.
- Disinfection of the puncture area.
- Sterile wiping of the puncture area - repeat this "spraying + wiping" procedure.
- Disinfect the puncture area again + allow to act (RKI Cat.1B).
- Put on sterile gloves.
- Deflate the port needle with NaCl 0.9%.
- Palpate the port chamber and fix the port with two fingers.
- Have patient look in the opposite direction.
- Hold the port needle securely
- Remove needle guard and puncture perpendicular to the membrane of the port until the needle stops.
- Open the clamp of the port needle.
- Aspiration test, if not possible only flush with io ml NaCl 0.9%.
- Then apply dressing with fixation.

5.2.4 Administering infusions

5.2.6 Removal of port needle *(excerpt from guidelines)*
- For longer length of stay, change needle every 5 days.
- Flushing the port with io ml NaCl 0.9%
- Secure the port with two fingers, grasp the port needle and pull.
- Safely dispose of port needle in designated drop
- Skin disinfection and dressing of the puncture site with sterile wound plaster
- Record in patient's chart.

It is recommended to flush the port catheter system with a saline solution every 3 months if it is not used for a longer period of time to prevent occlusion

Fig. 12.3 (continued)

Chirurgische Klinik

Abteilung für Allgemein-, Viszeral-,
Unfallchirurgie und Poliklinik

Prof. Dr. Dr. h. c. mult. M. W. Büchler
Geschäftsführender Direktor

Chirurgische Ambulanz
Leiter: Oberarzt Dr. med. Roland, Hennes
Sekretariat: Fon +49(0) 6221
566216
                          Fax +49(0) 6221 564637

Ambulanz   Fon + 49(0) 6221
566220
                          Fax + 49(0) 6221 567531
                          Ltg + 49(0) 6221
5639691

Patienten

Aufkleber

Sehr geehrte Kollegen,

wir haben Ihrer Patientin/ Ihrem Patienten

heute am ....

ein intravenöses Kathetersystem implantiert:

O Hochdruck-Port 6,6 F   O einen Hickman-Katheter   O einen zentr. Vorhofkatheter zur Hämodialyse

O Hochdruck-Port 8,0 F
                                                                  O dopellumig O einlumig

                                                                  Alle Katheter sind CT oder MRT - geeignet

Die **Implantation** erfolgte über:

O V. cephalica   O links   O durch Venae sectio

O V. subclavia   O rechts   O durch Punktion / Seldinger Technik

O V. jugularis externa

O V. jugularis interna

Sollte bei der Patientin / dem Patienten aktuell Hinweise auf eine Beeinträchtigung der körpereigenen Abwehr vorliegen (z.B. durch Erkrankungen bzw. oder durch Chemotherapie, o.ä.), empfehlen wir eine prophylaktische Antibiose für 3 bis maximal 5 Tage. Ein Rezept über

.... wurde von uns ausgestellt

Zur Schmerzbehandlung rezeptierten wir ....

Wir bitten Sie um regelmäßige Wundkontrollen, bei Infektionszeichen bitten wir um Rücksprache bzw. bitten Sie um Wiedervorstellung. Ebenso stehen wir auch bei allen anderen Problemen durch den Katheter wie z.B. V.a. Thrombosen, Funktionsstörungen usw. selbstverständlich jederzeit zur Verfügung. **Portsprechstunde jeden Donnerstag 13:30 – 15.30 Uhr**
Tel-Nr.: 06221 566220

O Die Haut wurde durch **Hautkleber** verschlossen, d.h. eine Entfernung von Hautfäden wird nicht erforderlich.
O Die Haut wurde durch **Naht** verschlossen, d.h. wir bitten um Entfernung des Nahtmaterials nach 10 – 14 Tagen.
O Die Haut wurde durch **resorbierbaren Faden** verschlossen, d.h. eine Entfernung des Nahtmaterials ist nicht notwendig.
O Wir empfehlen eine Portnadel mit der Länge: 19, 25 oder 38 mm. (bitte einkreisen)

Wenn nicht unbedingt erforderlich, sollte das Kathetersystem zunächst einige Tage (3-5) noch nicht benützt werden. Während Therapiepausen sollte der Port alle 6-(8) Wochen mit Kochsalzlösung gespült werden. Die Punktion des Ports darf nur mit Spezial-Nadeln (sog. Huber- oder Port-Nadel) vorgenommen werden. Bitte denken Sie auch zu einem späteren Zeitpunkt bei unklarem Fieber immer an eine mögliche Infektion des Ports.

Fig. 12.4 "Port letter": Patient and physician information on port installation. (Heidelberg University Hospital)

Evidence of Port Care

13

Reinhart T. Grundmann

Summary Evidence-based statements on port care are a rarity; most recommendations are based on empiricism. The most important measure in port care is compliance with hygiene guidelines. Only suitable special cannulas may be used for puncture. To reduce the risk of thrombosis and infection, blood sampling from the central venous line should be avoided. Ports should be flushed before and after fluid infusion or injection. There is no evidence for the type and amount of flushing solution, but usually only sterile saline is recommended for flushing and saline without added heparin may also be recommended for blocking the port.

13.1 Guidelines

13.1.1 Recommendations of the Robert Koch Institute

The Robert Koch Institute (RKI) recommends for the prevention of vascular catheter-associated infections (2002):

Puncture of the Port and Connection of Infusion Systems
- Before removing any existing dressing, hygienic hand disinfection must be performed (category IB).
- The puncture site must be disinfected over a large area, observing the prescribed contact time of the disinfectant (category IB).
- Sterile gloves must be worn for the puncture, which involves palpation and fixation of the port chamber between the palpating fingers (category IB).
- Only suitable special cannulas may be used (category IB).

R. T. Grundmann (✉)
DIGG of the DGG, German Society for Vascular Surgery and Vascular Medicine, Burghausen, Germany
e-mail: kontakt@medsachverstand.de

© Springer-Verlag GmbH Germany, part of Springer Nature 2022
R. Hennes, G. Müller (eds.), *Port Care*,
https://doi.org/10.1007/978-3-662-64494-2_13

- Aseptic connection of the infusion system (category IB).
- No recommendation on the maximum laying time of port needles (category III).

Dressing/Bandage Change of Port Systems
- With port needle connected, proceed as for central venous catheters.
- "Dormant" port systems, i.e. not in use, do not require a dressing (Category IB).

Laying Time of Port Systems
Average port catheter laying times of 240–315 days are reported in the literature. Reasons for port system removal may include end of therapy measures, unmanageable complications including refractory infections, irreversible catheter displacement, or damage or dislocation of the system.

Unmanageable complications require removal of the port system. Immediate removal of the port system in case of damage or dislocation (category IB).

13.1.2 DGEM Guideline

The S3 guideline of the German Society for Nutritional Medicine (DGEM) recommends (Bischoff et al. 2013a):

- For home parenteral nutrition (HPE) via a port system, port needle changes should be performed every 3–7 days for daily parenteral nutrition. [B; strong consensus]
- For intermittent feeding via a port system, the cannula should be removed for the non-infusion period. [Clinical consensus point (CCP); strong consensus].
- In the context of HPE, unused catheter or port systems should be flushed with isotonic NaCl solution before and after PE application. [CCP; strong consensus]. Solutions containing heparin should not be used for this purpose. [B; strong consensus].
- To reduce the risk of thrombosis and infection, blood sampling from the central venous line should be avoided. [strong consensus].
- As a first measure for blockages of catheter or port systems used for HPE, isotonic NaCl solution should be instilled. [CCP; strong consensus]. If this is unsuccessful, thrombolytics may be used for blockages after blood sampling. [C; strong consensus].
- When catheter infection is suspected in HPE, the first step should be to obtain blood cultures peripherally and from each catheter lumen. [CCP; Consensus]. Considering the clinical situation, systemic and intraluminal antibiotic therapy should be attempted if possible after antibiogram. [B; Consensus].
- The CVC should be removed if there are pronounced local or systemic signs of infection (incipient organ failure) and/or evidence of catheter-induced bacteremia with problem germs (e.g., Candida albicans, Pseudomonas strains, or Staphylococcus aureus). [B; Consensus].

- In problem patients, infection prophylaxis with antimicrobial agents (lock therapy) may be considered. [C; Consensus].

13.1.3 Australian Guideline (Queensland) (2015)

Flushing and Blocking of Ports
- The optimal volume and frequency of flushing and/or blocking ports for intermittent use (injections or infusions) is unclear. Until further evidence is available, clinical users should refer to the manufacturer's recommendations for flushing volume.
- Only single-dose solutions should be used.
- Clinical users should only use syringes with a diameter of a 10 ml syringe (or larger). Smaller diameter syringes may generate higher pressures in the lumen and cause catheter rupture.
- Clinical users should flush pulsatile (press-pause or start-stop-start).

Flushing Ports
- Flushing is recommended to promote and maintain openness and to prevent mixing of incompatible drugs and solutions.
- Sterile 0.9% saline solution for injection should be used to flush a port unless the manufacturer recommends flushing with a heparin saline solution.
- Ports should be flushed immediately by clinical users.
  - after implantation,
  - before and after fluid infusion or injection (since an empty infusion container lacks infusion pressure, allowing blood to flow back into the catheter lumen),
  - before and after blood sampling.
- Irrigation fluid and intervals should be documented by the clinician in the patient record.

Blocking Ports
Blocking means instillation of a solution to prevent occlusion when the device is not in use.

- There is insufficient information on what is the most appropriate solution to block a port. Primarily, heparinized saline has been used due to the anticoagulant properties of heparin. However, complications such as heparin-induced thrombocytopenia (HIT), altered coagulation status, and bleeding have been reported, especially when other anticoagulant treatment has been pursued. In addition, heparin is incompatible with some substances in solution, e.g., gentamycin sulfate.
- Until further evidence exists, clinical users should use 5 ml of sterile heparinized saline (10 units in 1 ml) to block a port that is no longer used for continuous infusion, with a view to future use—unless the manufacturer recommends that the catheter lumen be blocked with another solution.

- Ports that are not used should be flushed and blocked by a clinician every 4 weeks.
  - The most important measure of catheter blockage is the mechanical action of the measure as such, designed to prevent backflow of blood into the catheter tip.
- Low-dose oral warfarin or other systemic anticoagulants should not be prescribed for prophylaxis of catheter occlusions.

13.2 Overviews

13.2.1 Flushing and Blocking of Ports

A systematic literature review on flushing and blocking of central venous catheters has been prepared by Goossens (2015). According to this, the evidence of all recommendations is very low. At least 10 ml of 0.9% NaCl solution should be used for flushing, and the amounts of fluid used for blocking depend on the catheter volume. Overall, this overview shows that the Australian guideline (Sect. 13.1.3) has probably best translated the current state of knowledge into recommendations.

13.2.2 Management of Venous Port Systems in Oncology

A systematic review on evidence-based management of venous port systems was published in 2008 (Vescia et al.), which is still up-to-date due to the few studies published on the topic since then. Key statements are:

Access
- The port system is accessed via a special, non-punching Huber needle. The silicone membrane must be punctured vertically to avoid bending the tip. Strict aseptic precautions must be taken (sterile gloves, skin disinfection). A 2% chlorhexidine solution has been shown to be most effective in reducing catheter-associated infections; however, 70% alcohol, tincture of iodophor or tincture of iodine may be used alternatively.
- The needle can be left in place for 72 h, but should be replaced after 24 h if it has been used to administer blood products or lipid emulsions.
- When using a non-punching Huber needle, more than 2000 punctures are possible.

Infections
- Catheter-induced infections are facilitated by:
  - Contamination during implantation [of the port] (can be avoided by strictly aseptic technique)
  - Contamination of the catheter hub by introduction of substances from the outside, the most common route of infection in port systems

Table 13.1 Conditions for catheter/port removal or preservation for catheter-associated infections (According to Vescia et al. 2008)

Catheter preservation possible if all conditions are met	Catheter removal necessary
Absence of local signs of infection	Local complications such as port infection
Sterile blood cultures	Recurrent infection during/after antibiotic treatment
Clinically stable patient	– Clinically unstable patient
	– Persistent sepsis/bacteremia
	– Certain microorganisms: Staphylococcus aureus/ Candida species

- – Contamination of the infusion
- – Hematogenous from remote areas
- The most common pathogens of catheter-associated infections are coagulase-negative Staphylococci, Staphylococcus aureus and Candida species.
- If catheter-associated infection is suspected, aerobic and anaerobic blood cultures should be taken in pairs, via a peripheral vein and via the central catheter.
- In the case of a catheter-associated infection, the port system does not have to be removed in every case; the conditions for retention or removal are shown in Table 13.1.
- If catheter-induced infection is suspected, initiation of empiric antibiotic treatment is required, which is started before the results of the bacteriological examination are available.
- The so-called antibiotic block (Bouza et al. 2002) should be reserved for special situations in which recurrent infections occur despite aseptic conditions, but is not considered a routine method.

Thrombosis Prophylaxis

None of the studies performed to date has been able to demonstrate that routine prophylactic anticoagulation can prevent catheter-induced thrombosis in tumor patients with venous catheters.

13.2.3 Antibiotic Lock

The Infectious Diseases Society of America has issued clinical practice guidelines that comment, among other things, on antibiotic block for catheter infections (Mermel et al. 2009). It states:

- Antibiotic block is indicated for patients with long-term catheters for catheter-associated bloodstream infection (CRBSI) in whom catheter preservation is the goal in the absence of signs of exit or tunnel infection.

- In CRBSI, antibiotic block should not be used alone. Instead, the block should be used in conjunction with systemic antimicrobial treatment, with use of both regimens for 10–14 days.
- The residence time of an antibiotic block solution should generally not exceed 48 h before the block solution is reinstilled. In outpatients with femoral catheters, reinstitution should be performed every 24 h; in patients with dialysis catheters, the block solution can be renewed after each dialysis.
- Catheter removal is recommended for CRBSI due to S. aureus and Candida species in lieu of antibiotic block treatment and catheter preservation unless unusual circumstances exist, such as no alternative catheter implantation site.
- In patients with multiple positive catheter-drawn blood cultures that grow coagulase-negative Staphylococci or gram-negative bacilli and concurrent negative peripheral blood cultures, antibiotic block therapy without systemic treatment can be given for 10–14 days.
- For vancomycin, the concentration should be at least 1000 times higher than the minimum inhibitory concentration of the micro-organism involved (for example 5 mg/ml).
- Antibiotic block solutions contain the desired antimicrobial concentration [concentrations are given in the guideline] and are usually mixed with 50–100 units of heparin or normal saline in a volume sufficient to completely fill the catheter lumen (usually 2–5 ml).

13.2.4 Taurolidine Block

No studies are available on taurolidine block specifically for port systems. Liu et al. (2013) found six randomized studies for a systematic review on the question of whether a taurolidine block can prevent catheter-associated bloodstream infections (CRBSI). In this meta-analysis, compared with other block solutions, taurolidine block was able to reduce CRBSI risk without severe side effects or generation of resistant bacterial strains. It was not possible to assess whether the risk of thrombosis, for example, was increased compared with a heparin saline solution due to the small study sizes. Overall, however, the study situation was described by the authors as uncertain due to inadequate study methodology and small numbers. Another systematic review compared different antimicrobial block solutions for the treatment of CRBSI (Vassallo et al. 2015). The authors concluded that taurolidine is more effective than a heparin solution in preventing CRBSI. However, the data on the treatment of CRBSI is insufficient to assess the value of taurolidine in the treatment of CRBSI.

Nevertheless, an Italian consortium (Pittiruti et al. 2016) concluded that taurolidine/citrate was the most promising antibacterial/antithrombotic block solution, with further studies to test the most effective and safe concentrations (common concentrations to date have been 1.35–2%).

13.3 Studies

13.3.1 Heparin vs. Saline for Port Blockage

In a randomized trial, Goossens et al. (2013) compared blocking a port with a physiological saline solution (398 patients) to heparin blocking (404 patients). Ports were flushed with 10 ml of saline at the end of intravenous therapy or 20 ml every 8 weeks if parenteral nutrition and blood components were administered and the port was not used. In the heparin group, additional blocking with 3 ml of heparin (100 units/ml) was performed after flushing. Primary study endpoint was the impossibility to aspirate blood with still easy common injection. Easy injection/impossible aspiration was observed in 109 (3.5%) of 3019 accesses in the saline group and in 115 (3.8%) of 3017 accesses in the heparin group. Overall, 20.4% of patients in the saline group and 19.1% of patients in the heparin group developed at least 1 episode of "easy injection/impossible aspiration." Bloodstream infections were seen in 2 patients (0.03/1000 catheter days) in the saline group and in 6 patients (0.10/1000 catheter days) in the heparin group (no significant difference). One patient in the heparin group experienced HIT.

The study was able to demonstrate the non-inferiority of saline blockage compared to heparin blockage.

A similar result had already been reported earlier by Bertoglio et al. (2012), albeit with an inadequate study design. They retrospectively compared two groups. In group A ($n = 297$), cancer patients had their ports blocked with heparin solution (10 ml/500 U heparin), while in group B $n = 313$ blocking was done with 10 ml normal saline. The follow-up period was at least 12 months. The authors saw no difference in port survival (free of failure due to occlusion events) between the two groups, from which they concluded that normal saline was equally effective as heparin solution in keeping ports open in the treatment of cancer patients.

13.3.2 Heparin Dosage for Port Blockage and Flushing

Rosenbluth et al. (2014) retrospectively examined two consecutive study periods in which oncology pediatric patients had their ports flushed and blocked monthly with either 5 ml heparin, 100 units/ml ($n = 86$), or 5 ml heparin, 10 units/ml ($n = 89$). Tissue plasminogen activator (tPA) consumption was chosen as a measure of thrombotic catheter complications. In the first group, 0.82 tPA interventions per 1000 port days were seen, whereas in the second group with low heparin dosing, 0.59 interventions per 1000 port days were seen (no significant difference). Differences in complication and infection rates were also not found, so the authors concluded that 10 units of heparin/ml would be sufficient for blocking port catheters and questioned whether heparin was needed for blocking at all.

How should ports be cared for after completion of a chemotherapy cycle in patients with malignancies if they are not used? This question was retrospectively addressed by Kefeli et al. (2009). After completion of chemotherapy, 59 patients had their ports flushed every 6 weeks with 3 ml of normal saline and 1000 units of heparin, while 30 other patients had their ports flushed every 4 weeks with 3.5 ml of saline and only 500 units of heparin. All patients were followed up for at least 1 year. Because no thrombosis or infection was seen in either group, the authors recommended extending the irrigation intervals to 6 weeks for practicality. However, the retrospective study design was not able to say anything about the dosing of heparin.

In fact, longer flushing intervals can probably be maintained when the port is not in use, although this has not been verified in a randomized trial (Kuo et al. 2005). Odabas et al. (2014) reported flushing intervals of significantly more than 3 months, which were equivalent to so-called frequent port care (every 3 months) in terms of complication rates. However, as the rate of thrombosis was somewhat lower with 3-monthly flushing, perhaps—not evidence-based—flushing at 3-month intervals is recommended.

13.3.3 Skin Disinfection during Port Care

Kao et al. (2014) retrospectively compared two patient collectives of carcinoma patients with venous port systems in whom a povidone (PVP) iodine solution ($n = 396$) and a chlorhexidine solution ($n = 487$) were used for skin disinfection before port puncture. The median follow-up in both collectives was 198 days. The target outcome was the rate of bloodstream infections. Gram-negative bacteria were the most common pathogens, with no differences in the two groups (0.404 episodes per 1000 catheter days in the iodine group, 0.450 episodes in the chlorhexidine group). However, bloodstream infections caused by Gram-positive pathogens were significantly less frequent after chlorhexidine disinfection (0.110 episodes per 1000 catheter days vs. 0.269 episodes per 1000 catheter days in the iodine group). Thus, in this study, the rate of Gram-positive bloodstream infections was significantly reduced using chlorhexidine disinfection of the skin before port puncture compared to the use of PVP-iodine solution. Yet, this did not have a significant effect on the incidence of bloodstream infections overall, as the majority of infections were induced by Gram-negative pathogens—and there were no differences between the two groups in this respect.

13.3.4 Extravasation/Paravasation

Extravasation during the operation of a venous port system is a complication that in the majority of cases is due to inexperienced handling and is therefore avoidable; technical problems with the port as such are a rarity. In one review, the incidence of extravasation during port use was reported as 3–6% (Kurul et al. 2002). Causes included catheter damage or breakage, port-catheter separation and catheter tip malposition. However, punctures outside the port membrane or needle position changes during infusion were the most common. The latter were caused by insufficient needle fixation during infusion or the use of inappropriate needles. Extravasation of chemotherapeutic agents can lead to serious complications, which is why only well-trained personnel should carry out these applications. Prior to infusion, catheter openness must be ensured by first aspirating blood. If extravasation occurs, the infusion must be stopped and a chest X-ray is advised.

13.3.5 Antibiotic Block

A prospective observational study of antibiotic block therapy for port-associated bloodstream infection (BSI) with coagulase-negative Staphylococci in 44 patients was reported by Del Pozo et al. (2009). The antibiotics used were vancomycin or teicoplanin. Administered to block the port system was 5 ml with a concentration of 2 mg/ml vancomycin or 10 mg/ml teicoplanin plus heparin (100 units/ml). The antibiotic block was renewed daily. In addition, systemic antibiotic therapy was given in just over half of the cases. Study endpoint was failure to eradicate BSI, recognizable by port removal or by positive blood cultures at the end of treatment with the same bacterial spectrum as before. Treatment was successful in 39 patients (88.6%), with a cumulative port survival rate of 100% in the teicoplanin group and 77% in the vancomycin group. In this study, antibiotic block with teicoplanin in combination with systemic antibiotic treatment was able to achieve 100% port survival. Ultimately, however, randomized trials are lacking to definitively assess the value of this approach.

13.4   Conclusion

Conclusion for clinical practice (adapted from Vescia et al. 2008):

1. Port Care:
    • Strict adherence to hygiene rules is essential
    • Use of non-punching needles
    • If the port is not used in the follow-up of carcinoma patients, 3-month intervals for port flushing are probably sufficient
2. Thrombosis:
    • No recommendation for routine prophylactic anticoagulation
    • In case of manifest thrombosis treatment with low molecular weight heparin
3. Infections:
    • Port or catheter removal not always necessary
    • Identification of the causative microorganisms by blood culture and/or culture from the catheter tip
    • Adequate antibiotic treatment

References

Bertoglio S, Solari N, Meszaros P, Vassallo F, Bonvento M, Pastorino S, Bruzzi P (2012) Efficacy of normal saline versus heparinized saline solution for locking catheters of totally implantable long-term central vascular access devices in adult cancer patients. Cancer Nurs 35: E35–E42

Bischoff SC, Arends J, Dörje F et al (2013a) S3-Leitlinie der Deutschen Gesellschaft für Ernährungsmedizin (DGEM) in Zusammenarbeit mit der GESKES und der AKE. Künstliche Ernährung im ambulanten Bereich. Aktuel Ernahrungsmed 38:e101–e154

Bouza E, Burillo A, Muñoz P (2002) Catheter-related infections: diagnosis and intravascular treatment. Clin Microbiol Infect 8:265–274

Del Pozo JL, García Cenoz M, Hernáez S, Martínez A, Serrera A, Aguinaga A, Alonso M, Leiva J (2009) Effectiveness of teicoplanin versus vancomycin lock therapy in the treatment of port-related coagulase-negative staphylococci bacteraemia: a prospective case-series analysis. Int J Antimicrob Agents 34:482–485

Department of Health. Queensland Government (2015) Guideline: totally implantable central venous access ports. www.health.qld.gov.au/__data/assets/pdf_file/0030/444486/icare-port-guideline.pdf

Empfehlung der Kommission für Krankenhaushygiene und Infektionsprävention beim Robert Koch-Institut (RKI) (2002) Prävention Gefäßkatheter-assoziierter Infektionen. Bundesgesundheitsbl—Gesundheitsforsch -Gesundheitsschutz 45:907–924

Goossens GA (2015) Flushing and locking of venous catheters: available evidence and evidence deficit. Nurs Res Pract 2015:985686

Goossens GA, Jérôme M, Janssens C, Peetermans WE, Fieuws S, Moons P, Verschakelen J, Peerlinck K, Jacquemin M, Stas M (2013) Comparing normal saline versus diluted heparin to lock non-valved totally implantable venous access devices in cancer patients: a randomised, non-inferiority, open trial. Ann Oncol 24:1892–1899

Kao HF, Chen IC, Hsu C, Chang SY, Chien SF, Chen YC, Hu FC, Yang JC, Cheng AL, Yeh KH (2014) Chlorhexidine for the prevention of bloodstream infection associated with totally implantable venous ports in patients with solid cancers. Support Care Cancer 22: 1189–1197

Kefeli U, Dane F, Yumuk PF, Karamanoglu A, Iyikesici S, Basaran G, Turhal NS (2009) Prolonged interval in prophylactic heparin flushing for maintenance of subcutaneous implanted port care in patients with cancer. Eur J Cancer Care (Engl) 18:191–194

Kuo YS, Schwartz B, Santiago J, Anderson PS, Fields AL, Goldberg GL (2005) How often should a port-a-Cath be flushed? Cancer Invest 23:582–585

Kurul S, Saip P, Aydin T (2002) Totally implantable venous-access ports: local problems and extravasation injury. Lancet Oncol 3:684–692

Liu Y, Zhang AQ, Cao L, Xia HT, Ma JJ (2013) Taurolidine lock solutions for the prevention of catheter-related bloodstream infections: a systematic review and meta-analysis of randomized controlled trials. PLoS One 8:e79417

Mermel LA, Allon M, Bouza E, Craven DE, Flynn P, O'Grady NP, Raad II, Rijnders BJ, Sherertz RJ, Warren DK (2009) Clinical practice guidelines for the diagnosis and management of intravascular catheter-related infection: 2009 update by the Infectious Diseases Society of America. Clin Infect Dis 49:1–45

Odabas H, Ozdemir NY, Ziraman I, Aksoy S, Abali H, Oksuzoglu B, Isik M, Civelek B, Dede D, Zengin N (2014) Effect of port-care frequency on venous port catheter-related complications in cancer patients. Int J Clin Oncol 19:761–766

Pittiruti M, Bertoglio S, Scoppettuolo G et al (2016) Evidence-based criteria for the choice and the clinical use of the most appropriate lock solutions for central venous catheters (excluding dialysis catheters): a GAVeCeLT consensus. J Vasc Access 17:453–464

Rosenbluth G, Tsang L, Vittinghoff E, Wilson S, Wilson-Ganz J, Auerbach A (2014) Impact of decreased heparin dose for flush-lock of implanted venous access ports in pediatric oncology patients. Pediatr Blood Cancer 61:855–858

Vassallo M, Dunais B, Roger PM (2015) Antimicrobial lock therapy in central-line associated bloodstream infections: a systematic review. Infection 43:389–398

Vescia S, Baumgärtner AK, Jacobs VR, Kiechle-Bahat M, Rody A, Loibl S, Harbeck N (2008) Management of venous port systems in oncology: a review of current evidence. Ann Oncol 19: 9–15

Index

A

AIO nutrient solution mix, 71, 75
Analgesia, 55, 72, 83
Antibiotic Block, 107, 108, 111
Antibody administration, 6
Apharesis, 6, 10
Apharesis ports, 10
Arm port, 8, 64
Assisted living, 70–71
Assumption of costs, 69

B

Bacteremia, 17, 104, 107
Basic hygiene, 13
Bathing, 55
Biofilms, 16, 42
Bleeding tendency, increased, 84
Blocking
    guidelines, 106
Blood sample, 22, 84
Blood transfusion, 22

C

Cachexia, 60, 79
Cannula s. port needle, 35
Care manager, 67–70, 74
Case management, 28, 67
Catheter removal, 107, 108, 111
Check valve, 50
Chemotherapy, 2, 6, 63, 87, 109
Chlorhexidine, 14, 17, 20, 106, 110
Compounding, 71
Consultation, 55, 59, 67, 76, 81
Contrast agent, 2, 6
Cytostatic therapy
    complications, 61

D

Decannulation, 38
Delegation to non-medical staff, 27
DGEM guideline, 104–105
Dialysis, 6, 10, 108
Discharge management, 67
Disinfectants, 2, 13–15, 17, 19–22, 34, 42, 51,
        74, 90, 103
Disinfection
    patient and family education, 42–43
    the puncture site, 75, 92
Disinfection times, 74, 75
Dislocation, 19, 60, 76, 82, 89, 93, 104
Documentation
    catheter position, 88
Dressing
    changes, 20, 32, 33, 42, 45–52, 85, 86, 89, 92
    material, 49–50
Drip rate
    in children, 87
Dual chamber port, 2, 11

E

Education of relatives, 42
Elastomer pumps, 59, 61–63
Emla ointment, 92
Exit site infection, 17
Expert standard, 31–44
Extravasations, 10–12, 35, 37, 59–64, 82, 93,
        110–111
    cytostatic, 61
    in obese patients, 82

F

Feeding pumps, 71, 72
Fibrin layer, 16

Fixation sutures, 7
Flush
    guidelines, 105
Foil dressing, 49, 51, 61, 93
Foreign body sensation, 55
Function test, 10, 57

G
Gauge, 22, 34, 38, 46, 47
Groin ports, 64

H
Hair in the puncture area, 52
Hand disinfection, 13–15, 18, 21, 22, 35, 37,
    38, 51, 84, 91, 103
Health Care Transfer Directive (HÜR), 28–29
Health insurances, 29, 67–70
Hematoma, 32, 50, 57, 82, 85, 93
Heparin block, 18, 32
Heparin dosage, 109–110
High pressure port, 2, 5, 6, 61
Homecare companies, 67–68, 70, 71, 74, 76
Home health care prescription, 66
Huber pin, 106
Hygiene
    outpatient care, 66, 67, 74
    patient and family education, 42
    RKI recommendations, 18–19, 37
Hygiene guidelines, 9, 42, 64, 83, 103

I
Implantation technique, 7
Infection
    pathogens, 16
    prevention, 18, 19, 23
    procedure for, 41–42
    routes, 16–18
Initial puncture, 2, 38, 54, 90
Intraoperative care, 53–57

L
Leakage, 12, 37, 60, 93
Legal situation, performance of port puncture
    by nursing staff, 25–29
Leukemia, 83, 84
Local anesthesia, 53, 82
Local anesthetic, 53, 82

M
Mechanical problems, 76
Mohrenheim pit, 7

N
NaCl solution, 19, 73, 104, 106
Non-touch technology, 19–22, 74
Nursing crisis, 28
Nursing home, inpatient, 70
Nursing service, outpatient, 70, 74, 76
Nutrient solution mixtures, 71, 72
Nutritional solutions, 2, 5, 6, 64, 71

O
Obesity, 79
Occlusion, 10, 12, 38, 76, 82, 93, 105, 106, 109
Octenidine, 14, 17, 20
Outpatient care
    dealing with complications, 5–12
    hygiene, 66, 67, 74
    pharmacy, 67–69
    standard of care, 74

P
Pain therapy, outpatient, 72
Parenteral feeding
    guidelines, 104
Patient education
    ambulatory care, 70
Patient information, 95
Patient's consent, 27, 67
Pharmacy, 67–69, 71
Physician's letter, 101
Pocket infection, 17
Port cannula, 32, 34, 35, 37, 38, 89, 90
Port catheter system
    complications, 2, 5–12
    definition, 1
    indications, 5–12, 41
    localization, 88
    monitoring, 20
    oncology, v, 5, 6
    port placement in children, 81, 87, 88
    structure, 5, 6
Port catheter tube, 60
Port chamber
    in children, 87
    fixation, 8, 19, 21, 80, 103

sizes, 35, 37, 88
tilted, 8
Port consultation, 98
Port implantation
    intraoperative complications, 54–55
Port infection s. infection, 2, 16, 17, 23, 31,
        41–42, 52, 64, 76, 107
Port information brochure, 95
Port needle
    in children, 93
    fixation, 22, 60–61, 75, 82, 86, 91, 93
    length of stay, 9, 36, 46, 61, 80, 81
    for parenteral nutrition, 80
    position control, 60
Port needle change
    frequency, 18
Port needle diameter, 64, 80
Port needle dressing, 49, 50
Port needle grinding, 48
Port needle length
    in cachectic patients, 79–81
    in obese patients, 60, 81–83
Port needle removal, 22
Port passport, 5, 22, 35, 42, 55, 82, 88
Port puncture
    in children, 87
    implementation by nursing staff, 25–27
    materials, 37, 74
    patient preparation, 34
Port system
    for cachexia, 79–81
    in children, 87
    in obese patients, 81–83
Positioning control, 38, 60
Postoperative care
    in children, 87
    consultation, 55–57
Pressure sores, 80, 81
Puncture sites, 19, 21, 22, 32, 37, 38, 50–52, 60,
        64, 76, 80, 82, 90, 103
Push-and-go technique, 20, 21, 38, 41, 62, 64
PVP iodine, 14, 17, 110

R
Remanence, 14
Risk of infection in systemic diseases, 83
Robert Koch Institute

levels of recommendation, 19
recommendations, 18, 31

S
Safety port pins, 45
Saline block, 18
Scleroderma, 85–86
Secretion, 32, 50, 76, 94
Sepsis, 17, 107
Shave, 52, 92
Showering, 51, 55, 93
Signs of infection, 20, 32, 36, 41, 50, 55, 89, 93,
        104, 107
Silicone catheter, 10
Silicone membrane, 7, 11, 38, 41, 60, 80, 106
Skin disinfection, 14–15, 17, 21, 22, 91, 92,
        106, 110
Skin flora, 16–18
Specialized outpatient palliative care (SAPV),
        70
Staphylococcus, 17, 104, 107
Surface disinfection, 15
Sweating, 17, 82
Systemic diseases, 83–86

T
Taurolidine block, 18, 42, 108
Teicoplanin, 111
Thrombocytopenia, 84, 85, 105
Thrombosis prophylaxis, 107
Training
    patients and relatives, 3, 64
Transition management, 67
Tumor cachexia, 81

V
Vancomycin, 108, 111

W
Weight fluctuations, 79
Wound care, 45–52
Wound healing disorders, 32, 40, 63, 94
Wound inspection, 32, 50

Printed in the United States
by Baker & Taylor Publisher Services